An Atlas of Investigation and Management
ANGINA

An Atlas of Investigation and Management

ANGINA

Ian J Sarembock MB, ChB, MD, FAHA, FACC, FSCAI
Professor of Medicine
Director, Center for Interventional Cardiology & Coronary Care Unit
Cardiovascular Division & Cardiovascular Research Center
University of Virginia Health System
Charlottesville, Virginia, USA

With contributions from:

Fadi M El-Ahdab, MD
Fellow
Cardiovascular Division
University of Virginia Health System
Charlottesville, Virginia, USA

David Isbell, MD
Fellow
Cardiovascular Division
University of Virginia Health System
Charlottesville, Virginia, USA

Michael Ragosta, MD, FACC, FSCAI
Associate Professor of Medicine
Director, Cardiac Catheterization Laboratories
Cardiovascular Division
University of Virginia Health System
Charlottesville, Virginia, USA

CLINICAL PUBLISHING

OXFORD

Clinical Publishing

an imprint of Atlas Medical Publishing Ltd
Oxford Centre for Innovation
Mill Street, Oxford OX2 0JX, UK

Tel: +44 1865 811116
Fax: +44 1865 251550
Email: info@clinicalpublishing.co.uk
Web: www.clinicalpublishing.co.uk

Distributed in USA and Canada by:

Clinical Publishing
30 Amberwood Parkway
Ashland OH 44805 USA

Tel: 800-247-6553 (toll free within US and Canada)
Fax: 419-281-6883
Email: order@bookmasters.com

Distributed in UK and Rest of World by:

Marston Book Services Ltd
PO Box 269
Abingdon
Oxon OX14 4YN UK

Tel: +44 1235 465500
Fax: +44 1235 465555
Email: trade.orders@marston.co.uk

A catalogue record of this book is available from the British Library

ISBN-13 978 1 904392 59 0
ISBN-10 1 904392 59 8

The publisher makes no representation, express or implied, that the dosages in this book are correct. Readers must therefore always check the product information and clinical procedures with the most up-to-date published product information and data sheets provided by the manufacturers and the most recent codes of conduct and safety regulations. The authors and the publisher do not accept any liability for any errors in the text or for the misuse or misapplication of material in this work.

Printed by T G Hostench SA, Barcelona, Spain

Contents

Preface

The purpose of this book, *Angina: An Atlas of Investigation and Management*, is to share with the readers an outline of the most important aspects of the epidemiology, natural history, pathophysiology, clinical evaluation, non-invasive detection and invasive assessment of angina pectoris, a common manifestation of ischemic heart disease. In addition, we review the important non-atherosclerotic causes of chest pain and articulate an overall approach to the management of chronic angina with respect to goals of therapy including strategies to control symptoms and the role of coronary artery revascularization.

Over the last century, cardiovascular disease (CVD) has burgeoned from a relatively minor disease worldwide to a leading cause of morbidity and mortality. By 2020 it is projected that CVD will surpass infectious disease as the world's leading cause of death and disability. The major factors impacting this include the projected 60% increase in population between 1990 and 2020, the increasing life expectancy as a result of improvements in public health and medical care that are reducing rates of communicable disease, malnutrition, and maternal and infant deaths and the economic, social, and cultural changes that have led to increases in risk factors for CVD. Chronic angina is traditionally recognized as the cardinal symptom or manifestation of coronary artery disease (CAD), and worsening angina symptoms signal progression of the underlying pathology. Angina is a clear warning sign of a potential myocardial infarction; approximately 50% of myocardial infarction patients have had preceding angina. Overall, angina presents a tremendous economic burden on the health care system, society, employers, patients, and their families.

According to the American College of Cardiology/American Heart Association (ACC/AHA) 2002 Guideline Update for the Management of Patients with Chronic Stable Angina, the goals of chronic angina management are two-fold: to reduce morbidity and mortality; and to reduce symptoms. Medical therapy and revascularization procedures, either coronary bypass grafting (CABG) or percutaneous coronary interventions (PCI), play important roles in achieving these goals. However, these treatment options have limitations and significant expense and many patients have anatomical features or co-morbid conditions that prevent their optimal implementation. Newer drugs and procedures, such as transmyocardial revascularization, enhanced external counterpulsation, and gene therapy, are all under investigation.

An undertaking of this magnitude needs the combined efforts of numerous individuals, and as editor of this atlas, I want to express my sincere gratitude to my contributing authors, each of whom made critically important contributions. They have worked diligently to meet the format requirements of this atlas, the concept of which entails a brief and highly structured text, supported by extensive graphics, flowcharts and tables and numerous photographs of both the clinical signs of disease and of corresponding underlying pathology. Flowcharts, checklists and algorithms have been used to summarize key facts, and present the reader with a rapid reference to the diagnostic process. Tables include all key data of diagnostic value. In addition, it has been a true pleasure working with the publishing team of this atlas. Their advice, enthusiasm and commitment to the project were critical to its success and are sincerely appreciated.

Ian J Sarembock

Abbreviations

ACC American College of Cardiology
ACE angiotensin-converting enzyme
ACS acute coronary syndrome
ADR adverse drug reactions
AHA American Heart Association
BMI body mass index
BNP brain natriuretic peptide
BP blood pressure
CABG coronary artery bypass grafting
CAD coronary artery disease
CCB calcium channel blocker
COPD chronic obstructive pulmonary disease
CRP C-reactive protein
CSA chronic stable angina
CT computed tomography
DENSE displacement encoding with stimulated echo
DES drug-eluting stent
DSE dobutamine stress ECHO
EBCT electron beam computed tomography
ECHO echocardiography
ED Emergency Department
EECP enhanced external counterpulsation
ETT exercise tolerance test
EKG electrocardiogram
FFR fractional flow reserve
GERD gastroesophageal reflux disease
GI gastrointestinal
HDL high-density lipoprotein
IHD ischemic heart disease
ISD ischemic sudden death
LAD left anterior descending (artery)
LAO left anterior oblique

LBBB left bundle branch block
LCA left coronary artery
LDL low-density lipoprotein
Lp(a) lipoprotein-a
LV left ventricle
LVEF left ventricular ejection fraction
MDCT multi-detector computed tomography
METS metabolic equivalent tasks
MI myocardial infarction
MRFP magnetic resonance first pass perfusion
MRI magnetic resonance imaging
MSCT multi-slice CT
PCI percutaneous coronary intervention
PET positron emission tomography
PPI proton pump inhibitor
PTCA percutaneous transluminal coronary angioplasty
QOL quality of life
RAO right anterior oblique
RCA right coronary artery
RV right ventricle
SCS spinal cord stimulation
SECP sequential external counterpulsation
SPECT single photon emission computed tomography
SSFP steady state free precision
STEMI ST segment elevation myocardial infarction
TENS transcutaneous electrical nerve stimulation
TIC time–intensity curves
TIMI Thrombolysis In Myocardial Infarction (risk score)
TMR transmyocardial laser revascularization
TTE trans-thoracic echocardiography
UA unstable angina
WHO World Health Organization

1

Angina pectoris: epidemiology, natural history, and pathophysiology

Fadi El-Ahdab, MD, and Michael Ragosta, MD

Introduction

The term 'angina' is from the Latin 'angere' meaning to strangle, and was first described by the English physician William Heberden in 1768. Angina pectoris refers to the predictable occurrence of pain or pressure in the chest or adjacent areas (jaw, shoulder, arm, back) caused by myocardial ischemia. Typically, angina occurs in association with physical or emotional stress and is relieved by rest or sublingual nitroglycerin. Chronic stable angina refers to an anginal condition that has been observed over time and has not changed in terms of the level of exertion leading to angina, its severity, or frequency. It is important to distinguish stable angina from the acute ischemic syndromes which also cause anginal chest pain.

Epidemiology

Angina pectoris is due predominantly to ischemic heart disease (IHD) from coronary atherosclerosis. IHD represents the leading cause of death in the United States (**1.1**), from several mechanisms including acute myocardial infarction (MI), fatal arrhythmia, and heart failure. Although IHD is a major cause of death, its most common manifestation is chronic stable angina. In several studies performed in Western countries, the prevalence of angina pectoris in middle-aged individuals is estimated to be between 4 and 12%[1-3]. The American Heart Association estimates that there are 16,500,000 patients with stable angina in the United States, and the reported annual incidence of angina among individuals more than 30 years

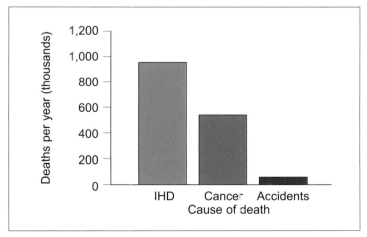

1.1 Causes of death in the United States per year (in thousands). Ischemic heart disease is the leading cause of death followed by cancer, cerebrovascular disease, and trauma.

old is 213 per 100,000 population. Angina pectoris is more often the presenting symptom of coronary artery disease (CAD) in women than in men, with a female-to-male ratio of 1.7:1. The frequency of atypical presentation is also more common among women compared with men. Women have a slightly higher mortality rate from CAD compared with men, in part because of an older age at presentation and a frequent lack of classic anginal symptoms, thus delaying the diagnosis and treatment of CAD.

Natural history

The majority of patients with chronic stable angina have underlying coronary atherosclerosis. The natural history of this condition is based on the extent, severity, and nature of the underlying atherosclerosis (*Table 1.1*). The majority of patients with angina remain stable, with predictable angina controlled with medical therapy or by limitation of activity. In some patients, the condition actually attenuates with reduction of angina over time (likely due to the development of collaterals) or even development of an asymptomatic state. The condition may exacerbate, however, with worsening of symptoms despite medical therapy and lead to substantial impairment in the quality of life from debilitating chest pain with minimal exertion. This may necessitate revascularization procedures such as percutaneous coronary intervention (PCI) or coronary bypass surgery. More importantly, the patient may develop an acute syndrome such as MI or unstable angina. The transformation of a stable to an unstable atherosclerotic lesion is poorly understood but is an important cause of death and morbidity in patients with coronary disease. It is interesting to note that while 50% of patients with acute MI have antecedent angina, few patients with angina progress to acute infarction. Two population-based studies from Olmsted County, Minnesota and Framingham, Massachusetts found 3–3.5% annual rates of MI in patients with angina[4,5]. Overall, survival in patients with chronic stable angina is good. The 5-year survival for patients with 'typical stable angina' was 83% in one study from Italy involving 519 patients with angina pectoris. Age, long-standing angina, the presence of previous infarction, heart failure, and an ischemic resting electrocardiogram (EKG) were among factors associated with a poor prognosis[6].

Table 1.1 Outcome of patients with coronary disease

- Chronic stable anginal pattern
- Exacerbation:
  - need for revascularization procedure:
    percutaneous coronary intervention
    coronary bypass surgery
  - development of acute coronary syndrome:
    acute ST segment myocardial infarction
    non-ST segment myocardial infarction
    unstable angina
- Improvement:
  - reduction in angina
  - development of asymptomatic state

Pathophysiology

The causes of angina pectoris are shown in *Table 1.2*. The most common cause of angina pectoris is coronary atherosclerosis, with a severe stenosis obstructing blood flow leading to myocardial ischemia (**1.2**)[7,8]. Other causes of angina due to obstruction are rare and include vasospasm, microvascular disease, coronary embolism, and anomalous coronary arteries. Angina can also be observed in the absence of coronary obstruction from decreased oxygen supply (anemia, hypoxemia, or profound hypotension) or from conditions causing increased oxygen demand (left ventricular hypertrophy, hypertensive crisis, or marked tachycardia).

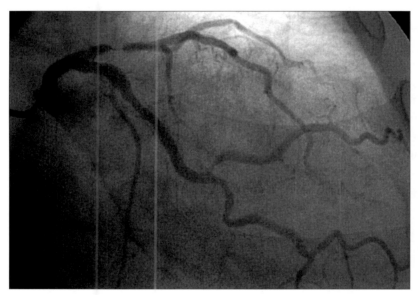

1.2 Angiogram of a patient with worsening chronic stable angina. It shows severe narrowing of the proximal left descending coronary artery secondary to atherosclerosis. This results in decreased perfusion pressure from the stenosis, mismatch in the oxygen demand–supply to the myocardium supplied by that artery, and consequently angina.

Table 1.2 Causes of angina pectoris

- Ischemia due to obstruction:
  - coronary atherosclerosis
  - coronary vasospasm
  - coronary emboli
  - anomalous coronaries
- Ischemia due to decreased oxygen supply:
  - anemia, hypoxia, hypotension
- Ischemia due to increased oxygen demand:
  - left ventricular hypertrophy, hypertension, tachycardia

The atherosclerotic coronary lesion is a lipid-containing plaque (also known as an atheroma) in the intima of the artery[7-11]. Atheroma formation is secondary to a complex set of mechanisms only partially understood, involving endothelial dysfunction, lipoprotein deposition and oxidation in the arterial wall, infiltration by inflammatory cells, cellular proliferation, especially smooth muscle cells, and matrix deposition (**1.3**). This mechanism may start at an early age. Endothelial dysfunction is thought to be the initial step in atherosclerosis (**1.4**). Endothelial dysfunction may result from the injurious effects of free radicals caused by tobacco smoking or from the effects of low-density lipoprotein (LDL) cholesterol, hypertension, diabetes, infectious agents, genetic factors, or a combination of these. Endothelial dysfunction results in increased endothelial permeability to lipoproteins, increased expression of adhesion molecules, and release of chemotactic factors that attract inflammatory cells (monocytes, macrophages, lymphocytes) and smooth muscle cells and facilitate their migration into the arterial wall. The fatty streak (**1.5**) results from the deposition of macrophages, lymphocytes, and smooth muscle cells into the arterial wall. In the arterial wall, macrophages containing LDL form 'foamy cells' and release cytokines and free radicals, causing more local damage and attracting more cells. As more foamy cells, inflammatory cells, and smooth muscle cells accumulate in the arterial wall, the fatty streak will grow in size and will tend to form a fibrous cap surrounding a lipid core (fibrofatty plaque or atheroma) (**1.6**). The cap consists of connective tissue and the lipid core includes foamy cells, leukocytes, and debris. As the plaque grows in size, it will push its way towards the lumen of the artery. When it is large enough to interfere with blood flow, ischemia and angina will result. Stable atheromas have a collagen-rich, thick fibrous cap, abundant smooth muscle cells, and fewer macrophages and usually result in chronic stable angina. Atheromas with thin caps, a large necrotic core and abundant macrophages tend to be less stable (vulnerable plaque) with a tendency to rupture, resulting in acute coronary syndromes, including MI.

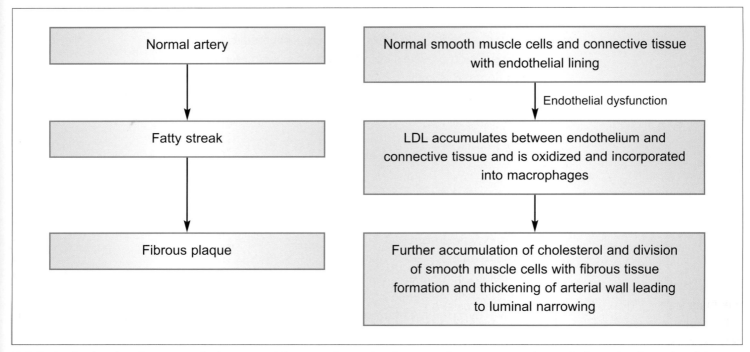

1.3 Steps in the development of atheroma. Atheroma formation is secondary to a complex set of mechanisms involving endothelial dysfunction, lipoprotein deposition and oxidation in the arterial wall, infiltration by inflammatory cells, cellular proliferation, especially smooth muscle cells, and matrix deposition.

1.4 Endothelial dysfunction leading to atherosclerosis. Endothelial dysfunction is thought to be one of the initial steps in atheroma formation. Endothelial injury from multiple causes (including elevated lipids, hypertension, and smoking) leads to increased permeability allowing the passage of lipoproteins and inflammatory cells into the artery wall. (From Ross, R. Atherosclerosis: an inflammatory disease. *NEJM*, 1999,**340**:115–126, with permission.)

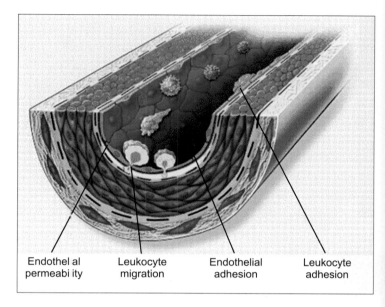

1.5 Development of a fatty streak. The fatty streak is formed when macrophages infiltrate the arterial wall and ingest oxidized lipids, predominantly LDL, to form 'foamy cells'. This is the earliest lesion in atherosclerosis and also contains scanty smooth muscle cells and other inflammatory cells such as lymphocytes. (From Ross, R. Atherosclerosis: an inflammatory disease. *NEJM*, 1999,**340**:115–126, with permission.)

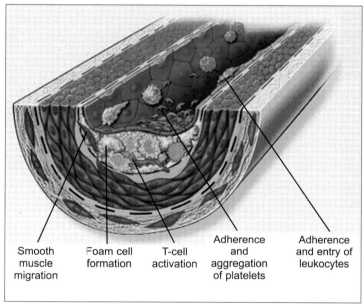

1.6 Development of an atheroma. This results from the accumulation of 'foamy cells', cellular debris, inflammatory cells including macrophages and mast cells, smooth muscle cells, and matrix, including collagen. Complex atheromas are usually organized into a necrotic core consisting mainly of lipid-rich 'foamy cells' and a fibrous cap containing smooth muscle cells and connective tissue. The morphology of the atheroma plays a major role in its stability. (From Ross, R. Atherosclerosis: an inflammatory disease. *NEJM*, 1999,**340**:115–126, with permission.)

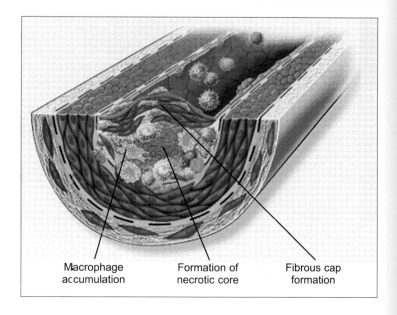

In patients with stable angina, the plaque tends to be slow growing and relatively stable. However, the plaque may undergo rapid and dynamic changes (**1.7**). Plaque rupture due to inflammation and other poorly understood mechanisms may result in platelet aggregation and thrombus formation. There are several consequences of this event. The event may be silent and lead to progression of luminal narrowing. More importantly, the thrombus may be occlusive and lead to sudden death from ventricular fibrillation or a nonfatal ST segment elevation MI. Nonocclusive thrombus may lead to significant flow limitation at rest and cause the acute ischemic syndromes of non-ST segment elevation MI or unstable angina. Unlike chronic stable angina, these conditions are potentially life-threatening and lead to substantial morbidity and mortality.

The mechanisms involved in the development of ischemia are complex and not solely related to the presence of a coronary stenosis. The amount of oxygen available in the myocardium is a function of the oxygen demand by the heart and of oxygen supply. Ischemia and subsequently angina result from mismatch between the amount of oxygen needed by the myocardium (oxygen demand) (*Table 1.3*) and the amount supplied to the myocardium (oxygen supply) (**1.8**). Myocardial oxygen demand is the major determinant of coronary blood flow. It is important to note that exercise may increase myocardial oxygen demand as much as 4–5-fold over baseline. Oxygen supply to the myocardium depends on coronary blood flow, the oxygen content of the blood (which depends on the blood oxygenation from the lungs and the amount of hemoglobin that carries oxygen), and the amount of oxygen extracted by the myocardium. Since the oxygen content is fixed and the myocardium already extracts most of the oxygen delivered to it, there is little or no oxygen extraction reserve. Thus, any increase in oxygen consumption requires an increase in coronary blood flow.

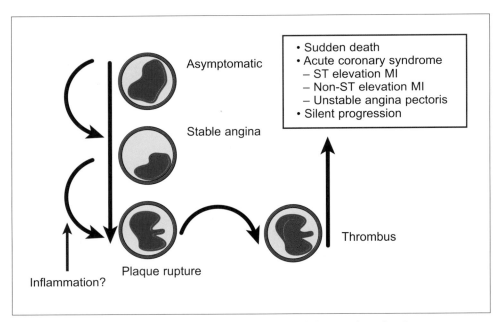

1.7 Pathogenesis of acute coronary syndromes. Atherosclerotic plaque may have a thick fibrous cap and be stable, causing chronic stable angina when flow-limiting. In contrast, it might have a thin fibrous cap, large necrotic core and abundant inflammatory cells, resulting in a vulnerable plaque that is prone to rupture, and thrombosis which might be occlusive (resulting in ST-elevation myocardial infarction or sudden cardiac death) or nonocclusive (resulting in an acute coronary syndrome). Causes of plaque rupture include inflammation and other unknown mechanisms.

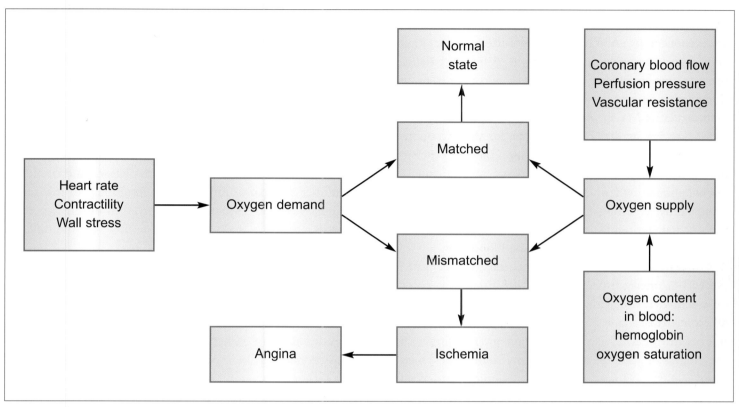

1.8 Determinants of myocardial oxygen supply and demand. Ischemia and subsequently angina result from mismatch between the amount of oxygen needed by the myocardium (oxygen demand) and the amount supplied to the myocardium (oxygen supply).

Table 1.3 Determinants of myocardial oxygen demand

- Wall stress (T = wall stress):

  $$\text{LaPlace's Law: } T \propto \frac{\text{pressure x radius}}{\text{wall thickness}}$$

- Heart rate
- Contractility

Coronary blood flow is determined primarily by the coronary resistance vessels (*Table 1.4*). These vessels in turn are influenced by endothelial-mediated factors, metabolites, and neurohormonal mechanisms. A complex balance of these factors maintains basal flow at fairly constant levels despite changing perfusion pressure, by a process known as 'autoregulation' (**1.9**). Autoregulation plays a major role in stabilizing myocardial blood flow under varying perfusion pressures and is stable over a large range of perfusion pressure. However, autoregulatory mechanisms are overwhelmed when the perfusion pressure drops significantly, resulting in a decrease in blood flow. Thus, myocardial ischemia represents an exhaustion of the compensatory mechanisms regulating blood flow.

Coronary flow reserve is an important mechanism that protects the heart from ischemia with progressive coronary obstruction (**1.10**). With progressive luminal narrowing from atherosclerosis, blood flow remains essentially unchanged at rest because of arteriolar vasodilatation and recruitment from the process of autoregulation until the stenosis becomes too severe (>80%). However, under hyperemic stress, the flow reserve is exhausted, and flow begins to decline when the diameter of the stenosis exceeds 50%.

Other factors may play a role in causing demand–supply mismatch and ischemia in patients with CAD. One suggested mechanism is paradoxical vasoconstriction of the diseased coronary vessels due to dysfunction of the coronary endothelium, which normally releases vasodilators such as nitric oxide. In atherosclerotic arteries, the dysfunctional endothelium fails to release vasodilators in response to hyperemia, resulting in vasoconstriction and ischemia. Another mechanism involves de-recruitment of myocardial capillary beds in diseased coronary vessels during hyperemic states, causing decreased blood flow to the affected myocardium.

Patients with chronic stable angina may have worsening of their symptoms due to progressive disease or transformation into an acute coronary syndrome. However, based on the complex mechanisms involved in the development of ischemia, factors other than progressive obstruction may be involved. These factors are summarized in *Table 1.5*.

Table 1.4 Determinants of coronary blood flow

- Driving pressure through the coronary vessel
- Extravascular compression
- Coronary resistance vessels:
  - endothelial factors – nitric oxide, prostaglandins, endothelin
  - metabolites – adenosine, hypoxia, hypercapnea
  - neurohormonal mechanisms

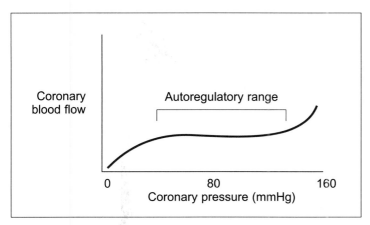

1.9 Autoregulation of coronary blood flow. The role of coronary autoregulation in stabilizing myocardial blood flow under varying perfusion pressures is important, and is stable over a large range of perfusion pressure. But when the perfusion pressure drops significantly, autoregulatory mechanisms become overwhelmed. This results in decrease in blood flow and subsequently ischemia.

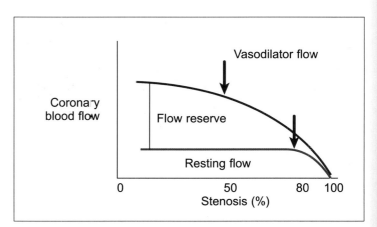

1.10 Relation of stenosis severity to coronary blood flow. Coronary flow reserve is an important mechanism that protects the heart from ischemia and generally increases from 2–5-fold with maximal coronary vasodilatation. Coronary flow reserve becomes diminished when lesions are >50% and is essentially overwhelmed for lesions >80%.

Table 1.5 Causes of myocardial ischemia other than coronary atherosclerosis

Increased oxygen demand
Noncardiac:
- Hyperthermia
- Hyperthyroidism
- Sympathomimetic toxicity (cocaine use)
- Hypertension
- Anxiety
- Arteriovenous fistula

Cardiac:
- Hypertrophic cardiomyopathy
- Aortic stenosis
- Dilated cardiomyopathy
- Tachycardia:
  - ventricular
  - supraventricular

Decreased oxygen supply
Noncardiac:
- Anemia
- Hypoxemia:
  - pneumonia, asthma, COPD, pulmonary hypertension, interstitial pulmonary fibrosis, obstructive sleep apnea
- Sickle-cell disease
- Sympathomimetic toxicity (cocaine use)
- Hyperviscosity:
  - polycythemia, leukemia, thrombocytosis, hypergammaglobulinemia

Cardiac:
- Aortic stenosis
- Hypertrophic cardiomyopathy

The exact mechanism(s) for the development of ischemic pain in patients with chronic stable angina is poorly understood. It is thought that myocardial ischemia results in the release of chemical mediators such as bradykinins and adenosine that stimulate nociceptors (**1.11**). The nociceptors then transmit the stimulus to the vagal and sympathetic afferent fibers in the heart. The afferent fibers transmit this signal to the thalamus and cerebral cortex via the spinal cord, leading to the sensation of pain.

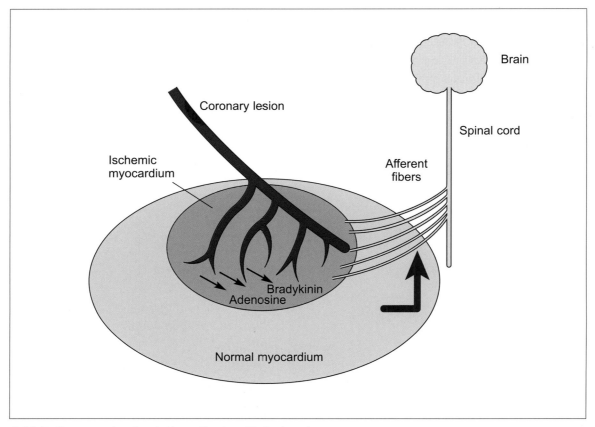

1.11 Pathogenesis of pain in patients with ischemia.

References

1 Reid DD, Brett GZ, Hamilton PJS, *et al.* Cardiorespiratory disease and diabetes among middle-aged male civil servants. A study of screening and intervention. *Lancet* 1974;1(7856):469–473.

2 WHO European Collaborative Group. Multifactorial trial in the prevention of coronary heart disease.1. Recruitment and critical findings. *Eur Heart J* 1980;1:73–80.

3 Shaper AG, Cook DG, Walker M, MacFarlane PW. Prevalence of ischemic heart disease in middle-aged British men. *Br Heart J* 1984;51:595–605.

4 Elveback LR, Connolly DC, Melton LJ III. Coronary heart disease in residents of Rochester, Minnesota 7. Incidence, 1950 through 1982. *Mayo Clin Proc* 1986;61:896–900.

5 Kannel WB, Feinleib M. Natural history of angina pectoris in the Framingham study. Prognosis and survival. *Am J Cardiol* 1972;29:154–163.

6 Brunelli C, Cristofani R, L'Abbate A. Long-term survival in medically treated patients with ischemic heart disease and prognostic importance of clinical and electrophysiologic data. *Eur Heart J* 1989;10:292–303.

7 Lambert CR. Pathophysiology of stable angina pectoris. *Cardiol Clin* 1991;9(1):1–10.

8 Zipes DP. Chronic coronary artery disease. In: RO Bonow, B Gersh, E Braunwald (eds), *Braunwald's Heart Disease: A Textbook of Cardiovascular Medicine*, 7th edn. Saunders, Philadelphia, 2005.

9 Crawford M, DiMarco J, Paulus W. *Cardiology*, 2nd edn. Mosby, St Louis, 2003.

10 Abrams J. Chronic stable angina. *NEJM* 2005;352:2524–2533.

11 Ross R. Atherosclerosis: an inflammatory disease. *NEJM* 1999;340:115–126.

Further reading

Lilly L. *Pathophysiology of Heart Disease*. Lippincott Williams & Wilkins, Philadelphia, 2002.

Angina pectoris: clinical evaluation

Fadi El-Ahdab, MD, and Michael Ragosta, MD

Introduction

The clinical evaluation of patients with chest pain is focused on deciding whether the patient's symptoms represent angina pectoris due to myocardial ischemia (2.1). This can usually be determined from a detailed history of the nature of the chest pain, an assessment of coronary artery disease (CAD) risk factors, and a focused physical exam. The probability of whether the patient has significant CAD and angina can be estimated as low, intermediate, or high. This 'pre-test' probability will direct the next step in the evaluation of the patient with chest pain and determine whether noninvasive, invasive, or no further testing is necessary. In general, low-risk patients do not undergo further testing but are counselled in risk-factor modification and followed up if necessary. Intermediate-risk patients generally undergo noninvasive testing, and high-risk patients most times proceed directly to coronary angiography.

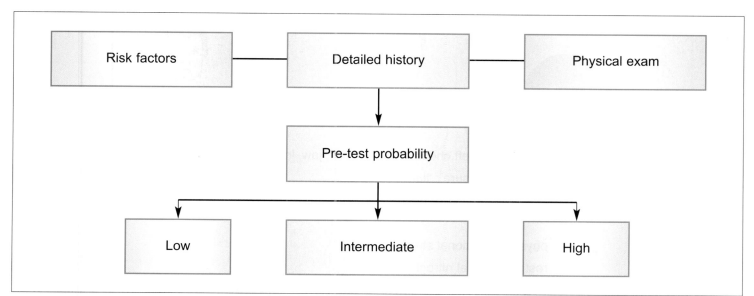

2.1 Clinical evaluation of patients with chest pain. A detailed history including risk factors for coronary atherosclerosis and a focused physical exam are the essential first steps in evaluating patients with chest pain. The next step is to determine the pre-test probability of the patient having angina. This will determine whether further testing is required and what type of test is needed.

2.2 Location of typical angina. Retrosternal chest pain radiating to the left arm is the most typical. Other locations suggestive of angina include jaw pain, epigastric pain, interscapular pain and right chest pain.

Classification of chest pain

Once a detailed history is obtained and the pain characteristics are identified, a classification of the chest pain into 'typical angina', 'atypical angina', or 'noncardiac chest pain' is helpful to direct the next steps in the evaluation of the patient (*Table 2.2*).

Table 2.2 Criteria for classification of chest pain

- Characteristic location, duration and quality
- Provoked by exertion or emotional stress
- Relieved by rest or nitroglycerin

Typical angina: meets all 3 criteria
Atypical angina: meets 2 criteria
Noncardiac pain: meets <2 criteria

History

The history is the most important step in the evaluation of patients with chest pain. It should include evaluation of the chest pain characteristics, history of CAD, and risk factors assessment. Characteristics of typical angina can be described using the mnemonic ANGINA-Dr (angina doctor) (*Table 2.1*). The location of typical angina is retrosternal, but it can also involve other areas like the epigastrium, left chest, arm, neck, jaw, or interscapular region (**2.2**). Pain above the mandible, below the epigastrium, or localized to a small area over the left lateral chest is rarely anginal. The quality of anginal pain is typically a 'heavy' sensation, a pressure or a tightness, and is often described as 'elephant on the chest', 'squeezing', or 'vise or grip-like'. Angina is less often described as burning or sharp pain. Angina is very unlikely when the pain is

stress, exposure to cold, or by other factors that increase the oxygen demand or decrease the oxygen supply to the heart. Stable angina is usually relieved by rest and/or sublingual nitroglycerin. Angina does not usually change with position, touch, respiration, or massage. The response to nitroglycerin is an important clinical clue and usually relieves stable angina within minutes. However, it should be remembered that esophageal spasm and other syndromes may also be relieved with nitroglycerin. A delay of more than 10 minutes before relief of chest pain is suggestive of either noncardiac pain or an acute coronary syndrome. There are a variety of associated symptoms. These include shortness of breath which usually results from significant myocardial ischemia causing elevation of the left ventricular end diastolic pressure, diaphoresis resulting from high

Case scenario

A 45 year-old Caucasian female presented to the Emergency Department (ED) with chest pain. The pain is located under her left breast. It is sharp in nature and has been waxing and waning on and off for 2 days. When the pain occurs, it lasts for several hours, is not associated with diaphoresis, nausea, or shortness of breath. The pain can occur at any time and is not clearly exacerbated by exertion. Sublingual nitroglycerin was given to the patient in the ED but it had no effect.

The patient's past medical history is significant for depression, anxiety, and tobacco smoking. She has no known family history of CAD. On physical exam, her blood pressure was 110/65, heart rate 90, respiratory rate 16. She is afebrile. Cardiovascular exam showed normal location of the apical impulse, normal heart sounds, a grade I/VI short systolic ejection murmur, and no gallop sound or friction rub. She has local tenderness under the left breast. Lungs were clear. Abdomen was soft with no masses or tenderness. Pulses were normal and symmetrical. No peripheral edema was present.

1 Based on the history and physical exam, what is the pre-test probability of CAD being the cause of this patient's chest pain?
A Low.
B Intermediate.
C High.
D Very high.

2 What's the next step in managing this patient?
A Send her home with no further testing.
B Stress test.
C Check EKG and cardiac enzymes.
D Coronary angiography.

3 EKG showed normal sinus rhythm, normal axis, no ST segment or T wave abnormalities. Cardiac enzymes were negative. What is the next step in this patient's management?
A Stress test.
B Send home to have follow-up with her primary care physician.
C Cardiac catheterization.
D CT of chest to rule out aortic dissection.

Answers

1 A

This patient's chest pain does not have the characteristic location or duration or quality of angina. It is not related to exertion and is not relieved by rest. Therefore, it is probably noncardiac chest pain (see *Table 2.2*). The patient has one major risk factor for CAD (tobacco smoking). The pre-test probability of this pain being angina is low.

2 C

The patient's pre-test probability of having angina is low. Ischemia, however, can sometimes have atypical presentations in some patients, especially females. An EKG and cardiac enzymes should be checked to rule out an acute coronary syndrome especially in light of the fact that her symptoms also occur at rest. Acute coronary syndromes include unstable angina and MI (ST elevation and non-ST elevation MI). The pathophysiology of acute coronary syndromes involves acute rupture of an atherosclerotic plaque in the coronary artery leading to platelet activation and thrombus formation, which may be occlusive (ST elevation MI) or nonocclusive (unstable angina or non-ST elevation MI). Acute coronary syndromes are associated with morbidity and mortality. This patient's presentation is unlikely to represent an acute coronary syndrome but an EKG and cardiac enzymes will add significant diagnostic and prognostic information. Stress test and coronary angiography may be indicated if she has evidence of ischemia on EKG or positive cardiac enzymes.

3 B

This patient has low pre-test probability of having myocardial ischemia. With the negative EKG and cardiac enzymes, the probability of having a major cardiac event is very low. It would be safe to send her home without further cardiac testing. Stress test is not indicated since it is difficult to interpret when the pre-test probability is low; cardiac catheterization is also not indicated since it is an invasive procedure and the yield from this test will be low, probably lower than the risks of performing the procedure. Further testing would be warranted if she has recurrence of symptoms. She should be counselled in the critical importance of smoking cessation together with lifestyle modification including diet, exercise, and weight loss.

References

1 Zipes DP. Chronic coronary artery disease. In: RO Bonow, B Gersh, E Braunwald (eds), *Braunwald's Heart Disease: A Textbook of Cardiovascular Medicine*, 7th edn. Saunders, Philadelphia, 2005.

2 Crawford M, DiMarco J, Paulus W. *Cardiology*, 2nd edn. Elsevier, Oxford, 2004.

3 Abrams J, Charlton G. *An Atlas of Angina*. Taylor & Francis Group, Oxford, 2002.

4 Becker R. *Chest Pain*. Butterworth-Heinemann Medical, Oxford, 2000.

5 Jackson G. *Angina*. Dunitz Martin, London, 2000.

6 Schofield P. *Angina Pectoris in Clinical Practice*. Dunitz Martin, London, 1999.

7 Kaski, JC. *Chest Pain With Normal Coronary Angiograms: Pathogenesis, Diagnosis, and Management*. Kluwer Academic Publishers, Boston, 1999.

8 Goldman L, Hashimoto B, Cook EF, Loscalzo A. Comparative reproducibility and validity of systems for assessing cardiovascular functional class: advantages of a new specific activity scale. *Circulation* 1981;**64**:1227–1234.

Chapter 3

Noninvasive detection of coronary artery disease

David Isbell, MD, and Ian J Sarembock, MB, ChB, MD

Introduction

The noninvasive detection of coronary artery stenosis continues to play a central role in the management of patients presenting with chest pain. In addition to identifying myocardial ischemia reliably, noninvasive techniques can assess disease severity, predict future clinical events, and even guide and monitor therapeutic interventions. As the prevalence of vascular disease continues to rise worldwide and there is a greater emphasis on rationing of healthcare resources, clinicians must be facile with the diagnostic modalities at their disposal. Those providers who understand the potential pitfalls and limitations of each noninvasive strategy and are adept at selecting patients appropriate for testing based on their pre-test probability will be most effective. Ultimately, there is no substitute for sound clinical judgement and all treatment decisions must be made with thoughtful consideration of test results in the appropriate clinical context.

Risk stratification in the Emergency Department

Electrocardiogram

While a 12-lead electrocardiogram (EKG) should be acquired in all patients presenting with chest pain, it may be completely normal in up to 50% of those with chronic stable angina and 5–10% of individuals with acute coronary syndromes (ACS). Prior EKGs should be used for comparison whenever possible and any changes noted. It is essential that serial EKGs are performed during observation, particularly if the patient was without chest pain during the initial recording. Where at all possible, an EKG should be obtained during active chest pain. Dynamic ST/T wave changes that occur with the onset of chest discomfort and improve with pain resolution are highly specific for unstable coronary disease. Several findings on resting 12-lead EKG predict the presence of coronary artery disease (CAD) (*Table 3.1*). Individuals with ST depression are at highest risk over the ensuing 6 months after the index event, perhaps because these patients tend to be older with a greater burden of ischemic disease (**3.1**). This analysis does not account for the one-third of patients with ST elevation myocardial infarction (MI) who die before arrival at a medical facility.

Table 3.1 Electrocardiogram findings predictive of underlying coronary artery disease

- ST elevation
- ST depression
- T wave inversion
- Pseudonormalized ST/T pattern
- Pathologic Q waves
- Left bundle branch block
- Atrioventricular block
- Ventricular tachycardia
- Atrial fibrillation
- Left ventricular hypertrophy

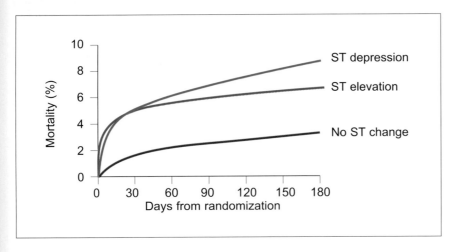

3.1 Predictive value of EKG: 6-month mortality based on electrocardiographic findings at presentation from the GUSTO IIb Acute Myocardial Infarction Trial. (Adapted from Savonitto S, *et al.* Prognostic value of the admission electrocardiogram in acute coronary syndromes. *JAMA* 1999;**281**:707–713.)

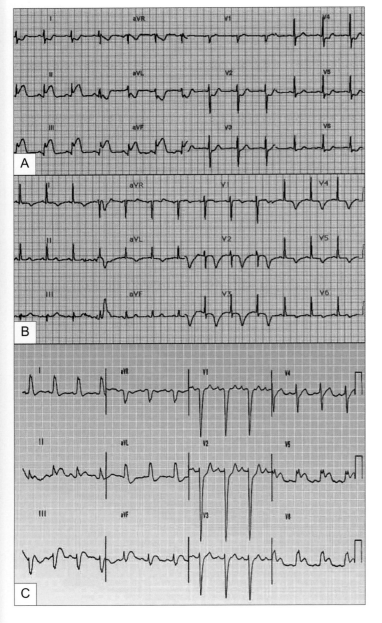

3.2 EKG presentations in acute ST elevation MI and acute coronary syndrome. **A**: In a patient presenting with acute onset of chest pain, this EKG pattern is consistent with an inferoposterior ST elevation infarct from complete occlusion of the RCA. ST depression in leads V2 and V3 with emerging R waves suggests involvement of the posterior wall, and hence a more extensive, and potentially lethal infarct. Acute reperfusion therapy would be warranted. **B**: This pattern of deep, symmetric anterior T wave inversion in V1–V3 (Wellens T waves) is highly suggestive of high-grade obstructive disease in the proximal LAD coronary artery. **C**: LBBB in a patient presenting with chest pain. In this instance, no prior EKGs were available for comparison. Concordant ST elevation in the anterolateral and inferior leads is consistent with an acute MI. This patient received thrombolytic therapy and had successful reperfusion. (Cardiovillage, permission obtained.)

Among patients presenting with an ACS, initial EKG findings are of critical importance. In addition to contributing to risk stratification, the EKG at initial presentation helps to guide subsequent management and even predict future clinical events including cardiovascular death[1]. Certain electrocardiographic patterns should be identified quickly and aggressive management instituted (**3.2**). Patients with left bundle branch blocks (LBBB) presenting with chest pain pose a unique diagnostic challenge as secondary ST/T wave changes at baseline are common. When there is clear evidence that the LBBB is new, aggressive therapy is almost always warranted. In patients presenting with old LBBB (or LBBB of unknown duration), the following criteria have been devised for diagnosing acute MI: (1) ST segment elevation of 1 mm or more that is concordant with the QRS complex, (2) ST segment depression of 1 mm or more in lead V1, V2, or V3,

(3) ST segment elevation of 5 mm or more disconcordant with the QRS complex[2]. A similar diagnostic strategy has been proposed for paced rhythms. In patients with nondiagnostic findings on EKG or LBBB patterns and symptoms consistent with cardiac chest pain, trans-thoracic echocardiography (TTE) may be used to detect regional wall motion abnormalities[3].

Serum markers

Several serum markers of myocardial necrosis have proven useful for both the diagnosis and prognosis of patients presenting with angina. Although all of these biochemical markers are released into the bloodstream after myocardial injury, they differ in their specificity for cardiac injury and the time course within which they are first detected, peak, and are cleared from the circulation (**3.3**). Cardiac troponins elevate relatively early and have the most

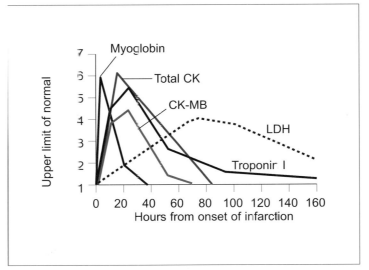

3.3 Biomarker kinetics in acute MI. Cardiac troponins have become the 'gold standard' and elevate relatively early and have the most favorable profile with respect to *both* sensitivity and specificity for myocardial necrosis, also providing prognostic information. (Adapted from Abbot Laboratories: www.abbottdiagnostics.com/Your_Health/Heart_Disease/ troponin-physicians-brochure.cfm.)

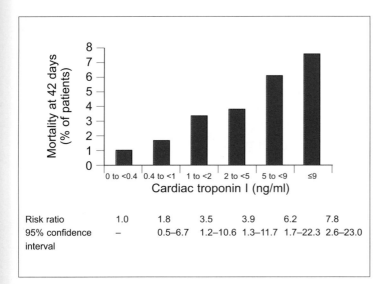

3.4 Prognostic value of troponin in acute coronary syndrome. There is a linear increase in risk of death at 42 days with progressive elevation of cardiac TnI, with the risk ratio increasing by 3.4-fold at TnI levels of 1–2 ng/ml and a further doubling of risk to 6-fold at TnI levels above 5 ng/ml. (Adapted from Antman EM, *et al*. Cardiac-specific troponin I levels to predict the risk of mortality in patients with acute coronary syndromes. *NEJM* 1996;**335**:1342–1349.)

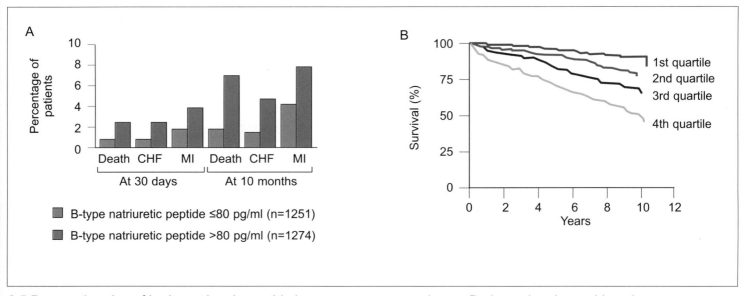

3.5 Prognostic value of brain natriuretic peptide in acute coronary syndrome. Brain natriuretic peptide, a hormone released from the myocardium in response to ventricular stretch, promotes vasodilation, increases urinary output, and inhibits the renin–angiotensin system. In patients with acute coronary syndromes, and in those with chronic stable angina, BNP levels have more recently been reported to predict adverse outcomes, including death, congestive heart failure, and MI. **A**: The incidence of death, new or progressive congestive heart failure (CHF), and new or recurrent MI at 30 days and 10 months among patients with BNP levels above, at, or below the pre-specified threshold of 80 pg/ml. *p*<0.005 for each comparison. **B**: Overall survival among patients with stable coronary artery disease, according to quartiles of NT-pro-BNP. The NT-pro-BNP levels were as follows: first quartile, <64 pg/ml; second quartile, 64–169 pg/ml; third quartile, 170–455 pg/ml; and fourth quartile, >455 pg/ml. *p*<0.001 by the log-rank test for the overall comparison among the groups. (Adapted from de Lemos JA, *et al*. The prognostic value of B-type natriuretic peptide in patients with acute coronary syndromes. *NEJM* 2001;**345**:1014–1021; Kragelund C, *et al*. N-terminal pro-B-type natriuretic peptide and long-term mortality in stable coronary heart disease. *NEJM* 2005;**352**:666–675.)

favorable profile with respect to *both* sensitivity and specificity for myocardial necrosis. Moreover, cardiac troponin levels provide prognostic information beyond that which can be obtained through standard clinical and electrocardiographic risk stratification[4] (**3.4**). Although highly specific for cardiac necrosis, troponin elevation is not the *sine qua non* of CAD, as other conditions may lead to cardiac injury and elevation of this enzyme.

Brain natriuretic peptide (BNP), a hormone released from the myocardium in response to ventricular stretch, promotes vasodilation, increases urinary output, and inhibits the renin–angiotensin system. In patients with ACS and in those with chronic stable angina, BNP levels have more recently been reported to predict adverse outcomes, including death, congestive heart failure, and myocardial infarction[5,6] (**3.5**). C-reactive protein (CRP) is an acute phase reactant produced in the liver in response to tissue injury and inflammation, and may play a direct role in atherosclerotic plaque formation and instability. High-sensitivity CRP assay can be utilized to predict subsequent events in patients presenting with ACS, and provide additional prognostic information beyond clinical predication tools and troponin levels[7] (**3.6**).

Imaging in the Emergency Department

Echocardiography

Inappropriately discharging patients with coronary ischemia from the Emergency Department (ED) can have devastating consequences. Patients discharged in the setting of acute infarction are generally younger, have less typical symptoms, and fail to manifest EKG evidence of ischemia. Furthermore, these individuals who are inappropriately discharged have increased mortality compared to those admitted to the hospital with MI[8]. Because of the serious implications of misdiagnosis, the incorporation of noninvasive imaging strategies to assist with early risk stratification has grown in popularity over the last 10–15 years. In the setting of a nondiagnostic electrocardiogram, two-dimensional echocardiography (ECHO) has been demonstrated to identify patients with CAD accurately in the ED[9]. Contrast ECHO, evaluating both regional function and myocardial perfusion, may enhance discriminatory power further and appears to provide additional prognostic information[10].

3.6 Prognostic value of high-sensitivity C-reactive protein in acute coronary syndrome. C-reactive protein is an acute phase reactant produced in the liver in response to tissue injury and inflammation and may play a direct role in atherosclerotic plaque formation and instability. High-sensitivity CRP assays can be utilized to predict subsequent events in patients presenting with acute coronary syndromes and provide additional prognostic information beyond clinical predication tools and troponin levels, as noted in these data from the CAPTURE trial of patients with refractory unstable angina. Predictive value for the end-point of mortality during the 6-month follow-up period according to both TnT and CRP status. (Adapted from Heeschen C *et al.* Predictive value of C-reactive protein and troponin T in patients with unstable angina: a comparative analysis. CAPTURE Investigators. Chimeric c7E3 AntiPlatelet Therapy in Unstable angina REfractory to standard treatment trial. *JACC* 2000;**35**:1535–1542.)

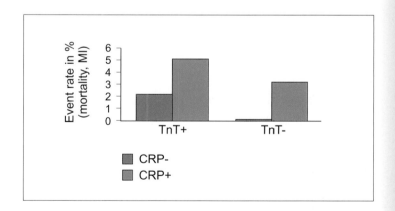

Nuclear

Several studies have also validated the use of resting radionuclide perfusion imaging performed in the ED among patients with anginal chest pain and a normal or nondiagnostic EKG[11–13]. This strategy clearly improves risk stratification and can reduce hospital admissions. In one study, 357 patients with symptoms suggestive of myocardial ischemia and a nondiagnostic EKG underwent Tc-99m tetrofosmin single photon emission computed tomography (SPECT) during or within 6 hours of symptoms[11]. Nuclear imaging accurately identified 18 out of 20 patients that went on to have a MI. Multiple logistic regression analysis demonstrated that SPECT imaging was a better predictor of outcomes than clinical data, and the excellent negative predictive value in this difficult population of patients could result in a mean cost saving of US$4,258 per patient.

Magnetic resonance and computed tomography

Both cardiac magnetic resonance imaging (MRI) and cardiac computed tomography (CT) are promising new techniques likely to revolutionize the way patients are evaluated and risk stratified in the ED presenting with chest pain. The diagnostic performance of cardiac MRI in patients presenting with chest pain appears promising. In one study evaluating 161 consecutive patients with a nondiagnostic EKG, MRI was more sensitive than strict EKG criteria ($p<0.001$), peak troponin ($p<0.001$), and the Thrombolysis In Myocardial Infarction (TIMI) risk score ($p=0.004$) and was more specific than an abnormal EKG ($p<0.001$)[14]. A subsequent study in 68 patients incorporated both rest and stress perfusion into the protocol[15]. Importantly, no adverse events were associated with administering vasodilator stress. Comprehensive cardiac MRI had a sensitivity of 96% and a specificity of 83% for the prediction of significant coronary stenosis, and was more sensitive and accurate than the TIMI risk score ($p< 0.001$).

Rapid diagnostic strategies incorporating electron beam computed tomography (EBCT) and multi-detector computed tomography (MDCT) have been encouraging. In one study of EBCT in patients presenting with chest pain to the ED and followed for 50 ± 10 months, the presence of coronary calcium and increasing score quartiles were strongly related to the occurrence of hard cardiac events and death[16]. MDCT using a 16-slice system has also been evaluated in patients presenting to the ED with chest pain[17]. Sensitivity and specificity for the establishment of a cardiac cause of chest pain were 83% and 96% respectively.

However, the real strength of the technique is its ability to identify both cardiac and important *noncardiac* causes of chest pain, including pulmonary embolism and aortic dissection.

Patient and test selection

Identification of patients who should undergo noninvasive testing and determining the appropriate test may be more challenging than interpretation of the results. Testing is most valuable in patients at intermediate risk for CAD, while those at very low and very high risk do not generally benefit. The rationale for this approach is derived from Bayes' Theorem, a method for determining the probability of an event by factoring in additional evidence and background information. In those ultimately selected for evaluation, decisions regarding whether or not the patient is a candidate for exercise and the method with which ischemia will be detected must be made. If exercise is deemed safe and the patient is capable, the exercise treadmill or bicycle is preferred over pharmacologically-induced stress in the majority of individuals. Both the workload achieved and hemodynamic response of the patient should be carefully documented. Local expertise and cost should also be taken into consideration when determining the best testing modality.

Exercise EKG stress testing

The exercise EKG test is simple, inexpensive, widely available, and well validated for use in identifying patients with CAD. Furthermore, EKG testing can help guide management and provides valuable prognostic information in a variety of clinical settings. The Duke Treadmill Score, which combines both exercise and EKG data, has been shown to predict long-term survival (**3.7**). The score is calculated as duration of exercise in minutes minus ($5 \times$ maximal ST segment deviation) during or after exercise minus ($4 \times$ the angina index). High-risk scores of <-10 give a 5-year survival rate of $<75\%$, while low-risk scores of $\geq +5$ give a 5-year survival rate of $\geq 95\%$[18].

A predictable series of pathophysiologic events transpires when cardiac metabolic demand exceeds myocardial oxygen delivery, such as caused by obstructive CAD. Nuclear imaging evaluates the earlier events of maldistribution of flow and hypoperfusion while stress ECHO assesses the later development of systolic dysfunction. It should be noted that EKG changes occur significantly later in the sequence of events compared to other measures of myocardial ischemia, and the symptom of chest pain is at the apex of the cascade (**3.8**). During exercise testing, changes in the ST/T wave segments with exertion are the most reliable signs of ischemia. However, specific attention must be given to the pattern and timing of ST/T wave changes as this can have important implications with respect to the sensitivity and specificity of the test (**3.9**). Note that downsloping ST depression is more predictive than horizontal ST depression, with upsloping ST depression being the least sensitive. Because diagnostic changes in the EKG may not occur until the post-exercise period, monitoring during recovery is mandatory (**3.10**). It is important to note that the ST depression does not localize to the anatomic region of ischemia.

3.7 Prognostic value of the Duke Treadmill Score. The score is based on exercise duration, severity of angina, and degree of ST depression. (Adapted with permission, Shaw LJ *et al*. Use of a prognostic treadmill score in identifying diagnostic coronary disease subgroups. *Circulation* 1998;**98**:1622–1630.)

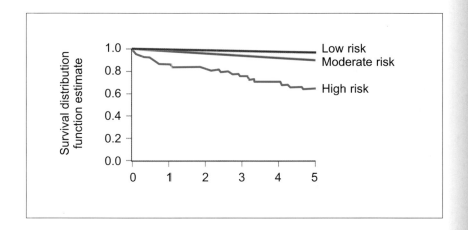

3.8 The ischemic cascade. The ischemic cascade represents a sequence of pathophysiologic events caused by obstructive coronary artery disease. Nuclear imaging evaluates the earlier events of maldistribution of flow and hypoperfusion while stress echocardiography assesses the later development of systolic dysfunction. It should be noted that EKG changes occur significantly later in the sequence of events and the symptom of chest pain is at the apex of the cascade. (Adapted from Schinkel AFL *et al*. Noninvasive evaluation of ischaemic heart disease: myocardial perfusion imaging or stress echocardiography? *Europ Heart J* 2003;**24**(9):789–800.)

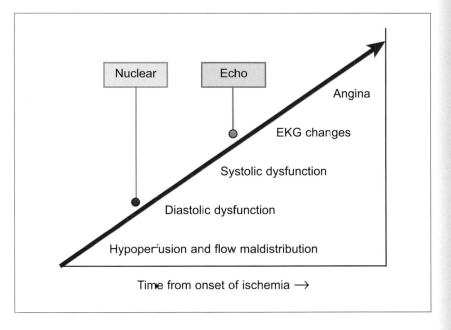

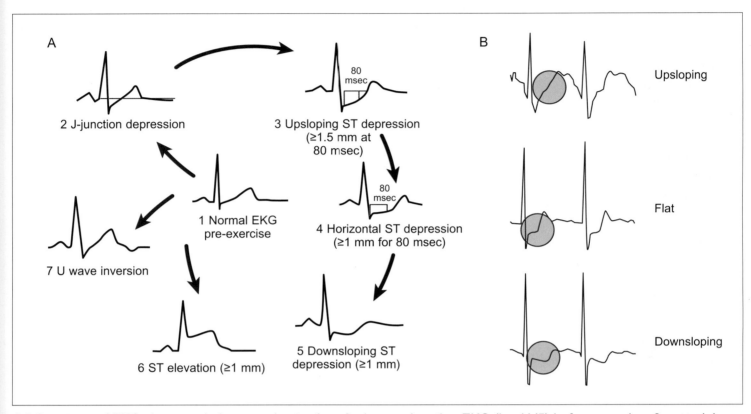

3.9 Spectrum of EKG changes during exercise testing. **A:** 1 normal resting EKG (lead V5) before exercise; 2 normal J point depression during exercise; 3 upsloping ST depression of subendocardial ischemia; 4 horizontal ST depression of subendocardial ischemia; 5 downsloping ST depression of subendocardial ischemia; 6 ST elevation caused by trans-mural ischemia; 7 U wave inversion. **B:** During exercise testing, electrocardiographic changes in the ST/T wave segments with exertion are the most reliable signs of ischemia. However, specific attention must be given to the pattern and timing of ST/T wave changes as this can have important implications with respect to the sensitivity and specificity of the test. Note that downsloping ST depression is more predictive than horizontal ST depression, with upsloping ST depression being the least sensitive. Because diagnostic changes in the EKG may not occur until the post-exercise period, monitoring during recovery is mandatory. It is important to note that the ST depression does not localize to the anatomic region of ischemia.

Exercise-induced ST elevation in leads devoid of Q waves is suggestive of severe, trans-mural ischemia or vasospasm. In contrast to ST depression, the lead location of the EKG changes does identify the distribution of the culprit lesion. In leads with pathologic Q waves, ST elevation most likely represents dyskinesis of infarcted segments, although it may represent injury current from viable myocardium within either the infarcted region or adjacent zones. In patients with anterior Q waves, nearly 50% will exhibit ST elevation during testing while only 15% of those with inferior Q waves will have this finding. ST segment elevation and depression in the same EKG denote more extensive ischemia.

Ventricular ectopy at rest in patients with a structurally normal heart generally carries a good prognosis[19]. However, the development of frequent ectopy either during exercise or immediately following predicts an increased risk of cardiovascular death[20] (**3.11**). In one study of 29,244 patients who were referred for stress testing, frequent ventricular ectopy developed in 7% of individuals, with 2% (589) occurring only during recovery. There was a strong correlation between ventricular ectopy only during the recovery period and subsequent death. Other studies have demonstrated that attenuated heart rate recovery following exercise predicts higher mortality independently of other factors, likely reflecting abnormalities in vagal tone[21].

Although considered quite safe, serious complications can occur with exercise testing and patients must be carefully screened (*Table 3.2*). When certain pre-existing

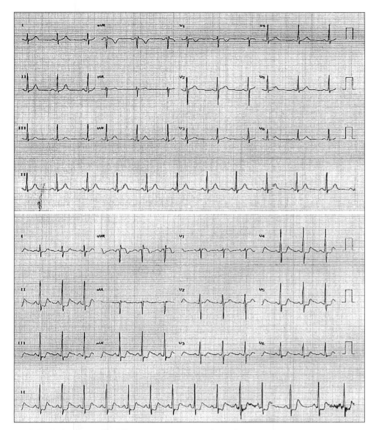

3.10 Ischemic EKG changes during the recovery period after treadmill exercise. EKGs from a patient both at rest and during exercise recovery. Note that no abnormalities were detected during exercise, yet early in recovery the patient developed chest pain and horizontal/downsloping ST depression diagnostic for ischemia. At catheterization a high-grade obstructive stenosis was observed in the mid-RCA.

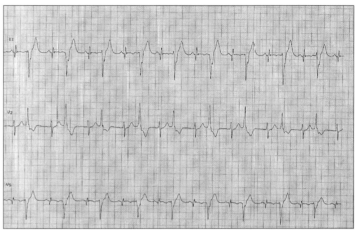

3.11 Ventricular ectopy during recovery after exercise treadmill testing. Ventricular bigeminy developed during recovery in a 55-year-old male following an otherwise normal treadmill test. Frequent ventricular ectopy developing either during exercise or in recovery is associated with a worse prognosis. If it develops in recovery, as in this example, it may be a sign of attenuated vagal reactivation and is associated with increased cardiovascular risk.

Table 3.2 Contraindications to stress testing

Absolute
- Acute aortic dissection
- Severe, symptomatic aortic stenosis
- Decompensated congestive heart failure
- Hemodynamically significant arrhythmias
- Acute myocardial infarction (48 hours)
- Active myocarditis

Relative
- Known left main coronary stenosis
- Severe, asymptomatic aortic stenosis
- Aortic aneurysm
- Recent stroke
- Severe, uncontrolled hypertension
- High degree heart block
- Hypertrophic cardiomyopathy with outflow obstruction

Note that there are absolute and relative contraindications to exercise stress testing. Clinical judgement should be used in the case of a relative contraindication and the exercise test should be carefully supervised by a physician

abnormalities in the resting EKG are identified (left ventricular hypertrophy [LVH], changes caused by digoxin, Wolff–Parkinson– White syndrome, resting ST/T changes, LBBB) the diagnostic value of the test is compromised (**3.12**) and techniques that do not rely on the EKG to detect ischemia are warranted, such as perfusion scan[22] (**3.13**).

Radionuclide imaging to detect ischemia

Nuclear imaging techniques have been employed for a number of years in the detection of hemodynamically significant coronary stenoses. Photons emitted from these isotopes following peripheral injection can be detected by specialized cameras designed to convert gamma rays into visible light. The most commonly used radioisotopes are thallium-201 (201Tl) and technetium-99m (99mTc). 99mTc is the preferred agent in many centers because it emits a higher energy photon and has a shorter half-life than 201Tl. This facilitates higher quality scans with fewer artifacts. Both tracers are distributed in relation to coronary blood flow and require viable cells for their uptake and retention. EKG gated acquisition of images enables the simultaneous analysis of both myocardial perfusion and left ventricular function (**3.14**). Adjunctive assessment of left ventricular function with perfusion enhances the detection of defects in multiple vascular territories in patients with severe three-vessel disease[23] (**3.15**).

A variety of strategies to induce myocardial stress or accentuate perfusion abnormalities can be used together with radionuclide imaging to detect coronary stenoses, although exercise testing is still the preferred modality when

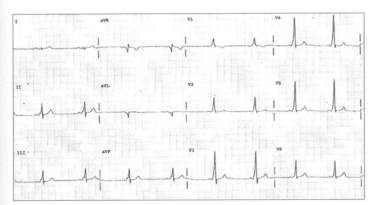

3.12 EKG tracing in pre-excitation syndrome. This EKG pattern is consistent with ventricular pre-excitation. Note the shortened PR interval, delta wave, widened QRS complex, and prominent R waves in the right precordial leads. As a consequence of pre-excitation, ST/T changes during exercise often do not reflect ischemia and a complementary imaging modality is warranted.

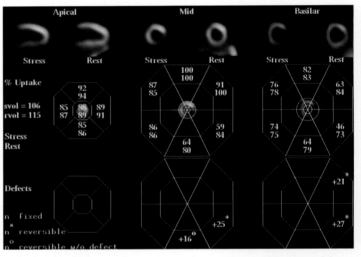

3.13 Myocardial perfusion imaging using technetium-99m sestamibi scan. End-systolic and end-diastolic gated images at the apex, mid-wall, and base are used to estimate regional wall thickening. Analysis is based on voxel counts rather than the detection of endocardial and epicardial borders and relies on the partial volume effect. Thickening fractions are then compared to values in a normal database and abnormal segments are flagged. In this example, note the reversible defect in the inferolateral wall of the left ventricle during exercise which redistributes at rest, consistent with inducible ischemia in the distribution of the RCA or possibly left circumflex artery.

feasible. *Table 3.3* presents the features found on radionuclide stress testing that infer high risk. Dobutamine increases myocardial oxygen demand through its potent chronotropic and ionotropic effects on the cardiovascular system, and can be administered intravenously prior to injection of the radiotracer. Side-effects with dobutamine infusion are frequent but rarely serious. Generally accepted end-points for dobutamine infusion include: >85% maximum predicted heart rate for age, systolic blood pressure (BP) >230 mmHg or diastolic BP >130 mmHg, a drop in systolic BP, onset of severe angina, sustained or

Table 3.3 High-risk features on radionuclide stress testing

- Large perfusion defect
- Multiple perfusion defects
- Stress-induced left ventricular dysfunction
- Transient cavity dilation
- Increased lung uptake (thallium)
- Resting left ventricular dysfunction

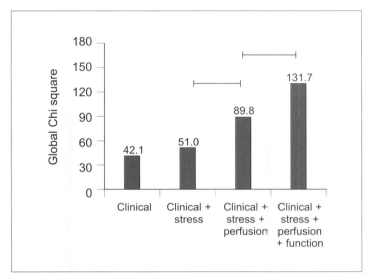

3.14 Incremental benefit of perfusion imaging and left ventricular function assessment in the detection of three-vessel CAD. The ability to predict three-vessel disease with Tc-99m sestamibi gated SPECT is significantly enhanced with the addition of left ventricular functional information to perfusion data. Multivariate logistic regression models for the prediction of three-vessel disease among all patients include a Chi square of 38.8 with 4 degrees of freedom, $p<0.0001$; Chi square of 41.8 with 2 degrees of freedom, $p<0.00001$. (Adapted from Lima RS, *et al*. Incremental value of combined perfusion and function over perfusion alone by gated SPECT myocardial perfusion imaging for detection of severe three-vessel coronary artery disease. *J Am Coll Cardiol* 2003;**42**(1):64–70.)

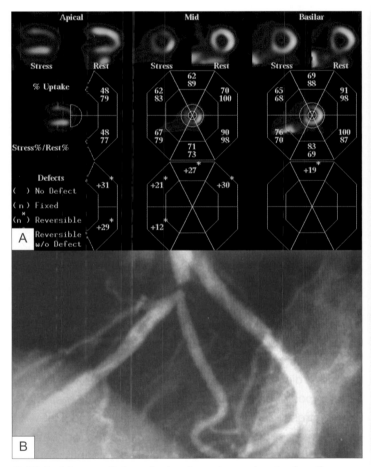

3.15 A: Myocardial perfusion imaging using technetium-99m sestamibi for the detection of inducible ischemia. In this example, there is extensive post-stress reversibility in the anterior, anteroseptal, and apical segments suggesting proximal disease in the LAD artery (defects are indicated by an asterisk). **B**: Cardiac catheterization confirmed high-grade obstructive disease in the proximal LAD.

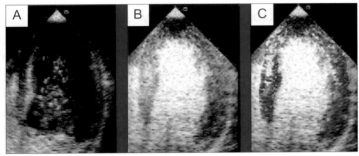

3.20 Improved endocardial border detection using myocardial contrast echocardiography. **A**: Ventricular myocardium at baseline, before LV contrast administration. **B**: Same view following LV contrast administration. Note the cavity of the left ventricle is opacified by the contrast agent. **C**: Following background subtraction. Note the dramatic improvement in endocardial border detection in **B** and **C** following contrast. The use of this technique can greatly enhance the detection of subtle wall motion abnormalities. (With permission from Lindner JL, Wei K. Contrast echocardiography. *Curr Prob Cardiol* 2002;**27**:454–519.)

Exercise stress ECHO

In comparison with standard exercise EKG stress testing, stress ECHO is superior in detecting CAD through visualization of regional abnormalities in left ventricular function during stress (**3.21**). The location and severity of inducible ischemia can be determined and valuable information regarding myocardial viability can also be obtained. ECHO is typically performed in conjunction with either exercise or dobutamine infusion. With treadmill exercise, continuous imaging is not feasible and it can be difficult to obtain appropriate windows immediately following completion of the protocol. Transient wall motion abnormalities induced during exercise may be missed and test sensitivity thereby reduced. To deal with this issue, many labs have implemented bicycle exercise protocols that facilitate continuous imaging. The sensitivity and specificity of exercise stress ECHO can be influenced by a number of factors including LBBB, severe hypertension, and prior MI with pre-existing wall motion abnormalities. The presence of LVH, which significantly influences exercise EKG testing, does not appear to influence the positive predictive value of exercise stress ECHO.

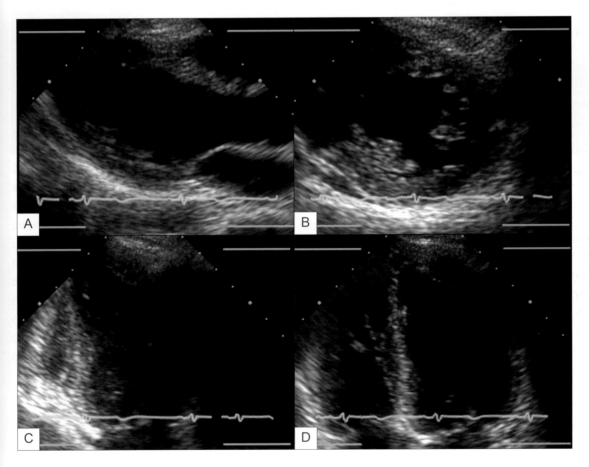

3.21 Wall motion abnormalities that develop during stress can be detected with transthoracic ECHO to identify regional myocardial ischemia. This figure represents four standardized views of the left ventricle that would be compared at both rest and during stress. **A**: two-chamber long axis; **B**: mid-ventricular short axis; **C**: two-chamber apical; **D**: four-chamber apical.

Dobutamine stress ECHO

Because of the technical difficulties often encountered while performing exercise stress ECHO, dobutamine stress ECHO (DSE) has grown in popularity. Through its potent ionotropic and chronotropic effects, dobutamine infusion increases myocardial oxygen demand and can provoke ischemia in patients with flow-limiting epicardial stenoses. As with exercise stress ECHO, ischemia is detected by a regional wall motion abnormality. The extent of wall motion abnormalities during stress predicts long-term outcome[24] (**3.22**). Atropine, which leads to increased hyperemia and partially counteracts the effects of underlying beta-blockade, can be administered if patients fail to reach 85% maximal predicted heart rate during dobutamine infusion.

ECHO detection of coronary stenosis at rest

In mid- to late systole, small myocardial arterioles collapse and blood contained in these vessels is displaced in a retrograde fashion into larger intramyocardial arteries[25]. Because of autoregulatory mechanisms, the blood volume in these arterioles and arteries is increased at rest in the presence of a hemodynamically significant coronary stenosis. High mechanical index myocardial contrast ECHO facilitates measurement of blood volume in these larger intramyocardial arteries during the cardiac cycle. In one study, measurement of arteriolar blood volume provided a sensitivity and specificity of 89% and 74%, respectively, for the detection of >75% stenosis[26]. The comparative advantages of stress ECHO and stress radionuclide perfusion imaging in the diagnosis of CAD are summarized in *Table 3.4*.

3.22 Predictive value of dobutamine stress echocardiography. Mortality of patients according to total extent of wall motion abnormalities (summed stress score) at peak stress. Through its potent ionotropic and chronotropic effects, dobutamine infusion increases myocardial oxygen demand and can provoke ischemia in patients with flow limiting epicardial coronary stenoses. As with exercise stress ECHO, ischemia is detected by a regional wall motion abnormality. The extent of wall motion abnormalities during stress predicts long-term outcome as illustrated on the right with 5-year mortality of 5–10% with single-vessel disease, 15% for 2-vessel disease and approximately 30% for 3-vessel disease. (Adapted from Marwick TH *et al*. Prediction of mortality by exercise echocardiography: a strategy for combination with the Duke treadmill score. *Circulation* 2001;**103**:2566–2571.)

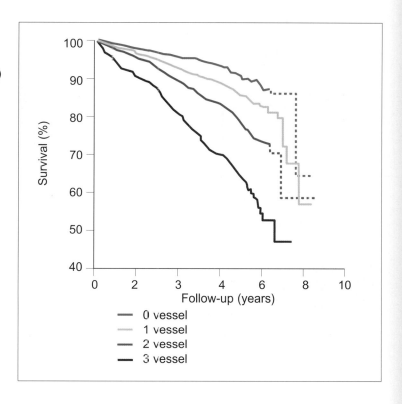

Table 3.4 Comparative advantages of stress echocardiography and stress radionuclide perfusion imaging in the diagnosis of coronary artery disease

Advantages of stress ECHO
- Higher specificity
- Versatility: more extensive evaluation of cardiac anatomy and function
- Greater convenience/efficacy/availability
- Lower cost

Advantages of stress perfusion imaging
- Higher technical success rate
- Higher sensitivity: especially for single-vessel coronary disease involving the left circumflex
- Better accuracy in evaluating possible ischemia when multiple resting left ventricular wall motion abnormalities are present
- More extensive published database: especially in evaluating prognosis

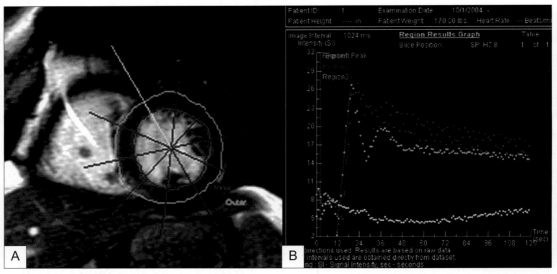

3.23 Magnetic resonance stress perfusion imaging with first pass of contrast and quantitative analysis. The myocardium is partitioned into sectors (**A**) and time intensity curves generated following injection of a gadolinium-based contrast agent (**B**). Regions subtended by a stenotic coronary artery have reduced perfusion following stress compared to normal regions, which is reflected in the diminished upslope of the time–intensity curve in that zone.

Magnetic resonance-based methods of detecting ischemia

MR perfusion

Currently employed radionuclide techniques are hampered by a limited spatial resolution, the potential risks of radiation exposure, and an inability to detect subendocardial perfusion defects reliably. Stress magnetic resonance first pass perfusion (MRFP) has generated a substantial amount of interest because of its favorable spatial resolution and safety profile when compared to both SPECT and PET[27]. MRFP is performed using a T1-weighted sequence to visualize a gadolinium-based contrast agent in transit through the heart and relies on the time–intensity curves (TIC). MRFP can be performed in a quantitative, semi-quantitative, or qualitative fashion (3.23). In clinical practice, qualitative analysis by an experienced clinician is generally performed and relies on the observer detecting regional differences in signal intensity over time (3.24).

3.24 Qualitative analysis of MRFP can also be performed and in experienced centers is a reliable method for detecting regions of ischemia. **A**: Short axis view through the mid-ventricle during stress imaging. **B**: Same location during rest perfusion imaging. In this example, notice the subendocardial perfusion abnormality during stress (arrows, **A**) compared to rest (**B**). This pattern is consistent with a high-grade stenosis of the RCA, which was later confirmed at coronary angiography.

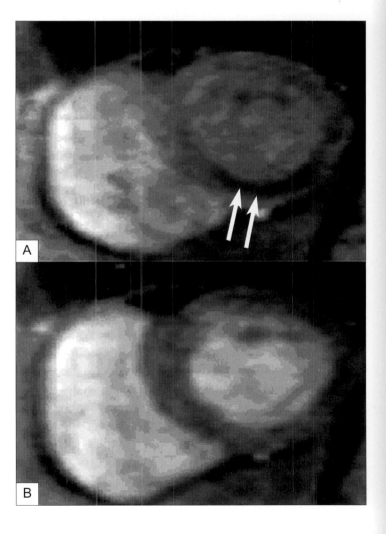

Dobutamine stress MR

The premise of dobutamine cardiac MRI is the same as with DSE: in a territory supplied by a stenotic coronary artery, blood flow is not available to compensate for increased metabolic demand, resulting in ischemia. This manifests visually as a segmental wall motion abnormality, which is a reliable sign of ischemia. The development of a regional wall motion abnormality precedes both angina and EKG changes. MRI has a number of potential advantages including improved visualization of all cardiac segments. Furthermore, new techniques that transiently embed tags within the myocardium enable improved detection of wall motion abnormalities and enable more sophisticated measurement of myocardial mechanics (**3.25**).

Coronary artery imaging using MRI is being pursued. Because the coronaries course along the epicardium in a layer of fat, fat saturation is an excellent tool for characterizing the coronary arteries. This technique is good at identifying the take-off of coronary arteries, and assessing the proximal portion of the vessels. However, diagnostic utility is limited in branch vessels and imaging remains very susceptible to artifacts from respiratory motion and cardiac arrhythmias (**3.26**).

Computed tomography

EBCT can noninvasively detect and quantify coronary artery calcification, an important marker of epicardial coronary stenoses[28]. EBCT acquires multiple, high-resolution axial slices through the heart which are gated to the EKG (**3.27A**). The absence of calcification detected on EBCT does have an excellent negative predictive value as lack of calcification is associated with <0.4% annual event rate. In patients with scores >100, the risk compared to the general population is increased 10-fold, while those with scores >400 will have 20 times the risk of cardiovascular events (**3.27B**, *Table 3.5*). However, the precise role of EBCT has yet to be defined as the presence of coronary calcium does not necessarily correlate with events, and patients without calcium may still be at risk for events from noncalcified, unstable plaques.

Multi-slice CT (MSCT) uses a multiple detector array that simultaneously obtains tomographic data at different slice locations and generates true isotropic voxels. Unlike EBCT, MSCT is contrast based and allows direct visualization of the coronary lumen. Currently, most centers employ either 16- or 64-slice systems, which allow for faster image acquisition, improved spatial resolution, and fewer

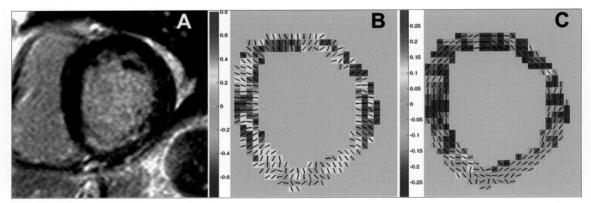

3.25 Magnetic resonance perfusion imaging with assessment of regional wall motion. Short-axis late gadolinium-enhanced inversion recovery gradient echo image in mid-diastole depicting subendocardial infarction in the inferior wall (**A**). **B**, **C**: First and second principal strain maps from SSFP (steady state free precision) cine DENSE (displacement encoding with stimulated echo) imaging. For first principal strain (**B**), orange and red represent normal strain and green indicates reduced strain. For the second principal strain (**C**), deep blue represents normal strain and green/yellow, abnormal strain. Note that the regions of abnormal strain extend well beyond the small zone of infarction.

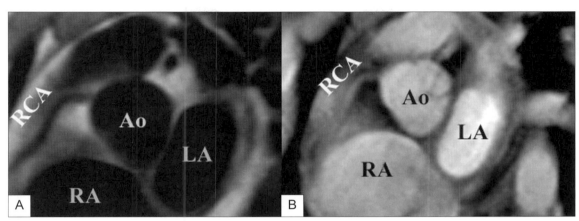

3.26 MR coronary artery imaging using 1.5 Tesla MRI scanner. Black blood, T1 turbo spin echo (**A**) gated to the cardiac cycle demonstrates the origin and course of the RCA in an individual where aberrant take-off of the RCA was a concern. T1 gradient echo with fat saturation (**B**) in the same orientation. RCA: right coronary artery; Ao: aorta; LA: left atrium; RA: right atrium.

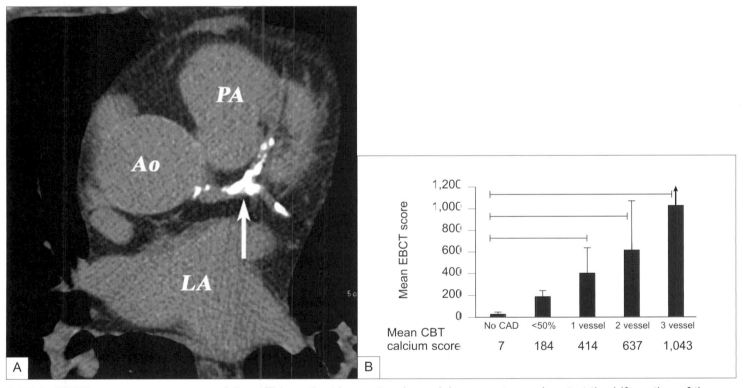

3.27 A: EBCT to assess coronary calcium. This patient has extensive calcium, most prominent at the bifurcation of the left main into the left anterior descending and circumflex systems (arrow). PA: pulmonary artery; Ao: aorta; LA: left atrium. **B**: EBCT calcium scores correlate with the extent of CAD as determined by angiography. Highest scores correlated with three-vessel disease; patients with nonischemic cardiomyopathy (no CAD or ≤50% by angiography) had the lowest calcium scores. (Adapted from Budoff MJ, *et al*. Ultrafast computed tomography as a diagnostic modality in the detection of coronary artery disease: a multicenter study. *Circulation* 1996;**93**:898–904.)

Two or more of the following?
1 Intermediate clinical predictors
2 Poor functional capacity
(<4 METS)
3 High surgical risk

No → No further pre-operative testing recommended

Yes ↓

Indications for angiography (e.g. unstable angina)?

Yes → Pre-operative angiography

No ↓

Patient ambulatory and able to exercise?*

Yes → Resting EKG normal?

Resting EKG normal? Yes → EKG / ETT

Resting EKG normal? No → Exercise echo or perfusion imaging**

No ↓

Bronchospasm?
II° AV block?
Theophylline dependent?
Valvular dysfunction?

No → Prior symptomatic arrhythmia (particularly ventricular tachycardia)?
Marked hypertension

Prior symptomatic arrhythmia... No → Pharmacologic stress imaging (nuclear or echo)

Prior symptomatic arrhythmia... Yes → Dipyridamole or adenosine perfusion

Yes ↓

Prior symptomatic arrhythmia (particularly ventricular tachycardia)?
Borderline or low blood pressure?
Marked hypertension?
Poor echo window?

No → Dobutamine stress echo or nuclear imaging

Yes → Other (e.g. Holter monitor, angiography)

3.29 Strategy for pre-operative assessment of CAD. Most patients with mild angina pectoris, particularly in the setting of poor functional capacity, require further testing. Unstable angina warrants cardiac catheterization.
* Can achieve >85% maximal predicted heart rate; ** in the presence of LBBB, vasodilator stress may be preferred.

catheterization, and 2-fold greater than a technetium-99m nuclear scan.

Not all patients are good candidates for MSCT. Those with fast or irregular heart rhythms, inability to cooperate with breathing instructions, renal insufficiency, and heavy vascular calcifications are poor candidates. Furthermore, patients must be aggressively beta-blocked and nitroglycerin administered prior to imaging to improve scan quality.

Special populations

As with men, cardiovascular disease is the leading cause of death among women[30]. Guidelines for the diagnosis and management of angina in women are the same as for men (**3.29**). However, important gender related differences must be acknowledged. Women are in fact more likely to present with atypical symptoms and in those with chest pain, noncardiac etiologies are not infrequent. Furthermore, women with CAD are generally older than their male counterparts and have less extensive coronary disease.

Exercise treadmill EKG testing is less predictive of CAD in women not only because the incidence of CAD is generally lower but also because patient selection is made more difficult by atypical presentations. As a consequence of breast artifacts, nuclear imaging is challenging and in some cases the discriminatory power of the test is compromised. In centers experienced with the technique, DSE may be the most reliable test in women with angina who are unable to exercise.

Patients with prior surgical revascularization and those with diabetes mellitus represent special subgroups that deserve further mention. In patients with coronary artery bypass grafting (CABG), the diagnosis of CAD has already been established and noninvasive techniques are most useful for guiding subsequent management. Individuals with vein grafts are at particularly high risk for future coronary events, and those presenting with acute coronary syndromes should be managed aggressively. Because baseline EKG abnormalities and LV dysfunction can make both exercise treadmill EKG and stress ECHO more difficult to interpret, myocardial stress perfusion imaging may be warranted in these patients, when available. In comparison with nondiabetics, patients with diabetes mellitus have more co-morbidities, greater disease burden, and worse long-term outcomes. Even among asymptomatic diabetics, the incidence of silent myocardial ischemia is as high as 20%[31].

In diabetics presenting with angina, the pre-test probability for disease is high and many may not be appropriate candidates for noninvasive stress testing.

Patients with angina scheduled to undergo noncardiac surgery can present a significant challenge. While unstable angina warrants surgical delay and aggressive intervention in almost all circumstances, the appropriate course of action for patients with more stable symptoms can be complicated. Careful consideration of the patient's symptom complex, exercise tolerance, and the nature of the operation can assist with guiding management. In many of these patients, supplemental noninvasive testing can provide valuable risk stratification prior to surgery. Patients with mild stable angina, good ventricular function, and a lack of high-risk features on noninvasive testing require no further intervention save beta-blockade. In contrast, unstable angina, angina unresponsive to medical therapy, and high-risk features on noninvasive testing typically warrant angiography.

References

1 Savonitto S, Ardissino D, Granger CB, et al. Prognostic value of the admission electrocardiogram in acute coronary syndromes. JAMA 1999;**281**:707–713.

2 Sgarbossa EB, Pinski SL, Barbagelata A, et al. Electrocardiographic diagnosis of evolving acute myocardial infarction in the presence of left bundle-branch block. GUSTO-1 (Global Utilization of Streptokinase and Tissue Plasminogen Activator for Occluded Coronary Arteries) Investigators. NEJM 1996;**334**:481–487.

3 Sabia P, Afrookteh A, Touchstone DA, Keller MW, Esquivel L, Kaul S. Value of regional wall motion abnormality in the emergency room diagnosis of acute myocardial infarction. A prospective study using two-dimensional echocardiography. Circulation 1991;**84**:I85–I92.

4 Antman EM, Tanasijevic MJ, Thompson B, et al. Cardiac-specific troponin I levels to predict the risk of mortality in patients with acute coronary syndromes. NEJM 1996;**335**:1342–1349.

5 de Lemos JA, Morrow DA, Bentley JH, et al. The prognostic value of B-type natriuretic peptide in patients with acute coronary syndromes. NEJM 2001;**345**:1014–1021.

6 Kragelund C, Gronning B, Kober L, Hildebrandt P, Steffensen R. N-terminal pro-B-type natriuretic peptide and long-term mortality in stable coronary heart disease. *NEJM* 2005;**352**:666–675.

7 Heeschen C, Hamm CW, Bruemmer J, Simoons ML. Predictive value of C-reactive protein and troponin T in patients with unstable angina: a comparative analysis. CAPTURE Investigators. Chimeric c7E3 AntiPlatelet Therapy in Unstable angina REfractory to standard treatment trial. *J Am Coll Cardiol* 2000;**35**:1535–1542.

8 Lee TH, Rouan GW, Weisberg MC, *et al.* Clinical characteristics and natural history of patients with acute myocardial infarction sent home from the emergency room. *Am J Cardiol* 1987;**60**:219–224.

9 Peels CH, Visser CA, Kupper AJ, Visser FC, Roos JP. Usefulness of two-dimensional echocardiography for immediate detection of myocardial ischemia in the emergency room. *Am J Cardiol* 1990;**65**:687–691.

10 Tong KL, Kaul S, Wang XQ, *et al.* Myocardial contrast echocardiography versus thrombolysis in myocardial infarction score in patients presenting to the emergency department with chest pain and a nondiagnostic electrocardiogram. *J Am Coll Cardiol* 2005;**46**:920–927.

11 Heller GV, Stowers SA, Hendel RC, *et al.* Clinical value of acute rest technetium-99m tetrofosmin tomographic myocardial perfusion imaging in patients with acute chest pain and nondiagnostic electrocardiograms. *J Am Coll Cardiol* 1998;**31**:1011–1017.

12 Varetto T, Cantalupi D, Altieri A, Orlandi C. Emergency room technetium-99m sestamibi imaging to rule out acute myocardial ischemic events in patients with nondiagnostic electrocardiograms. *J Am Coll Cardiol* 1993;**22**:1804–1808.

13 Wackers FJ, Lie KI, Liem KL, *et al.* Potential value of thallium-201 scintigraphy as a means of selecting patients for the coronary care unit. *Br Heart J* 1979;**41**:111–117.

14 Kwong RY, Schussheim AE, Rekhraj S, *et al.* Detecting acute coronary syndrome in the emergency department with cardiac magnetic resonance imaging. *Circulation* 2003;**107**:531–537.

15 Plein S, Greenwood JP, Ridgway JP, Cranny G, Ball SG, Sivananthan MU. Assessment of non-ST segment elevation acute coronary syndromes with cardiac magnetic resonance imaging. *J Am Coll Cardiol* 2004;**44**:2173–2181.

16 Georgiou D, Budoff MJ, Kaufer E, Kennedy JM, Lu B, Brundage BH. Screening patients with chest pain in the emergency department using electron beam tomography: a follow-up study. *J Am Coll Cardiol* 2001;**38**:105–110.

17 White CS, Kuo D, Kelemen M, *et al.* Chest pain evaluation in the emergency department: can MDCT provide a comprehensive evaluation? *Am J Roentgenol* 2005;**185**:533–540.

18 Shaw LJ, Peterson ED, Shaw LK, *et al.* Use of a prognostic treadmill score in identifying diagnostic coronary disease subgroups. *Circulation* 1998;**98**:1622–1630.

19 Kennedy HL, Whitlock JA, Sprague MK, Kennedy LJ, Buckingham TA, Goldberg RJ. Long-term follow-up of asymptomatic healthy subjects with frequent and complex ventricular ectopy. *NEJM* 1985;**312**:193–197.

20 Frolkis JP, Pothier CE, Blackstone EH, Lauer MS. Frequent ventricular ectopy after exercise as a predictor of death. *NEJM* 2003;**348**:781–790.

21 Cole CR, Blackstone EH, Pashkow FJ, Snader CE, Lauer MS. Heart-rate recovery immediately after exercise as a predictor of mortality. *NEJM* 1999;**341**:1351–1357.

22 Gibbons RJ, Balady GJ, Bricker JT, *et al.* ACC/AHA 2002 guideline update for exercise testing: summary article: a report of the American College of Cardiology/American Heart Association Task Force on Practice Guidelines (Committee to Update the 1997 Exercise Testing Guidelines). *Circulation* 2002;**106**:1883–1892.

23 Lima RS, Watson DD, Goode AR, *et al.* Incremental value of combined perfusion and function over perfusion alone by gated SPECT myocardial perfusion imaging for detection of severe three-vessel coronary artery disease. *J Am Coll Cardiol* 2003;**42**:64–70.

24 Marwick TH, Case C, Sawada S, *et al.* Prediction of mortality using dobutamine echocardiography. *J Am Coll Cardiol* 2001;**37**:754–760.

25 Chilian WM, Marcus ML. Phasic coronary blood flow velocity in intramural and epicardial coronary arteries. *Circ Res* 1982;**50**:775–781.

26 Wei K, Tong KL, Belcik T, *et al.* Detection of coronary stenoses at rest with myocardial contrast echocardiography. *Circulation* 2005;**112**:1154–1160.

27 Isbell DC, Kramer CM. Cardiovascular magnetic resonance: structure, function, perfusion, and viability. *J Nucl Cardiol* 2005;**12**:324–336.

28 Budoff MJ, Georgiou D, Brody A, *et al.* Ultrafast computed tomography as a diagnostic modality in the detection of coronary artery disease: a multi-center study. *Circulation* 1996;**93**:898–904.

29 Leber AW, Knez A, von Ziegler F, *et al.* Quantification of obstructive and nonobstructive coronary lesions by 64-slice computed tomography: a comparative study with quantitative coronary angiography and intravascular ultrasound. *J Am Coll Cardiol* 2005;**46**:147–154.

30 Mieres JH, Shaw LJ, Arai A, *et al.* Role of noninvasive testing in the clinical evaluation of women with suspected coronary artery disease: consensus statement from the Cardiac Imaging Committee, Council on Clinical Cardiology, and the Cardiovascular Imaging and Intervention Committee, Council on Cardiovascular Radiology and Intervention, American Heart Association. *Circulation* 2005;**111**:682–696.

31 Wackers FJ, Young LH, Inzucchi SE, *et al.* Detection of silent myocardial ischemia in asymptomatic diabetic subjects: the DIAD study. *Diabetes Care* 2004;**27**:1954–1961.

Further reading

Ellestad MH. *Stress Testing. Principles and Practice.* Oxford University Press, Oxford, 2003.

Feigenbaum H, Armstrong WF, Ryan T. *Feigenbaum's Echocardiography*, 6th edn. Lippincott Williams and Wilkins, Philadelphia, 2004.

Gibbons RJ. ACC/AHA/ACP-ASIM guidelines for the management of patients with chronic stable angina: executive summary and recommendations. A Report of the American College of Cardiology/American Heart Association Task Force on Practice Guidelines (Committee on Management of Patients with Chronic Stable Angina). *Circulation* 1999;**99**:2829–2848.

Zaret BL, Beller GA. *Clinical Nuclear Cardiology*, 3rd edn. State of the Art and Future Directions. Mosby, Philadelphia, 2004.

Coronary angiography and ancillary techniques for the invasive assessment of angina pectoris

Michael Ragosta, MD

Introduction

Selective coronary angiography is an invasive method for evaluating patients with angina pectoris syndromes. It is an important tool in determining the underlying cause of angina, especially in its ability to identify and quantify the presence of coronary artery disease (CAD). Since the first selective coronary angiogram performed by Mason Sones in 1959, coronary angiography has become commonplace, with over 1.5 million performed in the United States each year. Coronary angiography requires physician skill both in performance and in image interpretation and requires knowledge of the indications, contraindications, limitations, and potential complications of the procedure.

The procedural aspects are fairly simple. Arterial access is obtained most commonly from the femoral artery. Brachial or radial artery approaches can also be used. The operator chooses a pre-formed catheter to facilitate selective engagement of either the right or left main coronary artery. It is important for the operator to engage the coronary ostium selectively in a co-axial fashion to optimize image quality and reduce the risk of arterial injury from the catheter. Catheter choice depends on several patient variables including aortic root size and shape, aortic valve plane orientation, and the angle of coronary ostial origin. Typically, the right coronary artery (RCA) is selectively engaged with a right Judkins catheter (**4.1A**) and the left main coronary artery (LCA) with a left Judkins catheter (**4.1B**) under fluoroscopic guidance. These catheters are available in several sizes and, in addition, other catheter shapes are available to allow co-axial and selective engagement (**4.1C–E**). Once a catheter is selectively engaged, iodinated contrast is hand-injected into the artery while the operator acquires the radiographic images. It is important for the operator to image each arterial segment free of overlapping vessels with at least two views obtained 90 degrees apart. Most operators utilize several standard angiographic views. The arterial segments optimally imaged in these views are summarized in *Table 4.1*. An example of these views in a patient with normal coronary arteries is shown in **4.2**. These include left anterior oblique (LAO) and right anterior oblique (RAO) caudal and cranial views and lateral view.

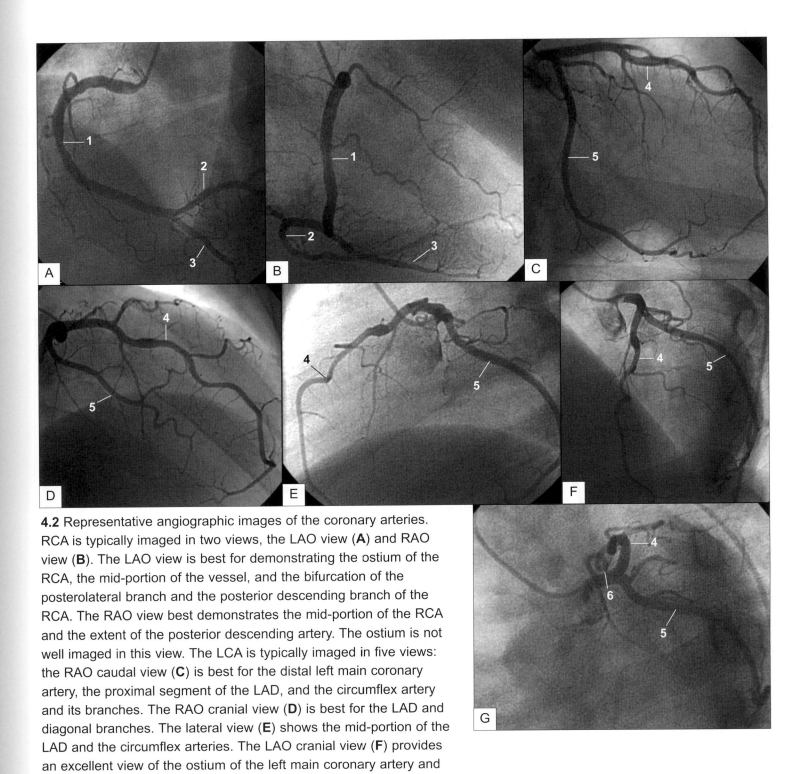

4.2 Representative angiographic images of the coronary arteries. RCA is typically imaged in two views, the LAO view (**A**) and RAO view (**B**). The LAO view is best for demonstrating the ostium of the RCA, the mid-portion of the vessel, and the bifurcation of the posterolateral branch and the posterior descending branch of the RCA. The RAO view best demonstrates the mid-portion of the RCA and the extent of the posterior descending artery. The ostium is not well imaged in this view. The LCA is typically imaged in five views: the RAO caudal view (**C**) is best for the distal left main coronary artery, the proximal segment of the LAD, and the circumflex artery and its branches. The RAO cranial view (**D**) is best for the LAD and diagonal branches. The lateral view (**E**) shows the mid-portion of the LAD and the circumflex arteries. The LAO cranial view (**F**) provides an excellent view of the ostium of the left main coronary artery and the origin of the diagonal arteries from the LAD. The LAO caudal view (**G**) is also known as the 'spider view', and is the best view for the distal left main stem and the proximal segments of the LAD, circumflex artery, and ramus intermedius branch. (1: RCA; 2: posterolateral branch of RCA; 3: posterior descending artery; 4: LAD; 5: left circumflex artery, marginal branch; 6: distal left main stem.)

Indications and contraindications

Angiography provides important clinical information about coronary anatomy and the presence of luminal obstruction in patients with angina pectoris, and is indispensable in guiding revascularization decisions (*Table 4.2*). It is important to note, however, that the angiogram does not inform the clinician about the relationship of a patient's chest pain syndrome to the presence of a coronary lesion observed on an angiogram. For example, a patient may undergo angiography for evaluation of a chest pain syndrome and be found to have co-existing coronary atherosclerosis, which may or may not explain the chest pain syndrome. Thus, clinical correlation is imperative for interpreting properly the findings on angiography.

Patients with angina pectoris may vary widely in terms of the extent of disease apparent on coronary angiography. There is no correlation between the extent of disease noted on angiography and symptoms. For example, the angiograms shown in **4.3** were obtained in a patient with minimal angina yet show extensive (three-vessel) coronary disease. Similarly, a patient may have severe, disabling angina with atherosclerotic narrowing involving only a small branch.

Table 4.2 Information provided by coronary angiography

- Coronary anatomy:
    - vessel dominance
    - vascular territories
    - anomalous vessels
    - coronary collateral circulation
- Coronary luminal obstruction:
    - guide revascularization decisions
- Coronary blood flow

Information not provided by coronary angiography
- Relation of chest pain to presence of coronary disease

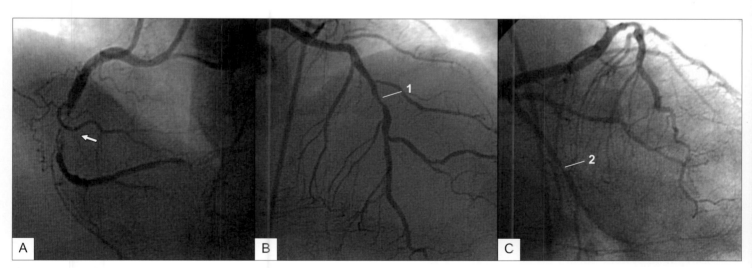

4.3 Angiography in a 70-year-old male for evaluation of a highly abnormal and 'high-risk' stress test with minimal angina pectoris on extreme exertion. Extensive luminal obstruction is noted in all three coronary arteries on angiography. **A**: RCA showing obstruction with collateralization of the distal vessel (arrow); there was severe narrowing of the mid-portion of the LAD (1) (**B**) and near occlusion of the mid-portion of the circumflex artery (2) (**C**). The patient was treated with bypass surgery.

Common indications for coronary angiography are summarized in *Table 4.3* and have been extensively addressed in practice guidelines[1]. In patients with ST segment elevation myocardial infarction (STEMI), coronary angiography is often performed during the acute stage to identify the culprit lesion and plan reperfusion therapy. Patients treated with lytic or medical therapy for STEMI or patients with other acute coronary syndromes (ACS) such as non-STEMI or unstable angina often undergo angiography for risk stratification assessment, in response to an abnormal noninvasive test or for the development of a complication such as recurrent ischemia, heart failure, or arrhythmia. Patients with stable angina may undergo angiography if they have an abnormal (especially 'high-risk') noninvasive test or if they are limited by symptoms despite medical therapy. Coronary angiography is also useful for evaluating patients with atypical chest pain syndromes with noninvasive tests that are either abnormal or nondiagnostic, particularly if pain is recurrent.

It is important to understand when coronary angiography is not indicated or is potentially harmful under certain circumstances (*Table 4.4*). Angiography should not be performed if revascularization is not an option either because the patient will not consent or has contraindications to surgical or percutaneous revascularization. Similarly, conditions which increase the risk of angiography should be addressed before proceeding. In such cases, the risk–benefit ratio should be carefully considered before proceeding with angiography.

Table 4.3 Indications for coronary angiography

- Management of patients with acute STEMI to identify and re-perfuse the infarct-related artery
- Management of patients with acute STEMI who have received lytic or medical therapy and have recurrent angina, heart failure, or arrhythmia or for risk stratification purposes
- Patients with non-STEMI or unstable angina in whom an invasive management strategy is chosen
- Evaluation of select patients with stable angina with or without a prior, abnormal noninvasive test
- Evaluation of certain 'high-risk' asymptomatic patients
- Patients with chest pain syndromes and abnormal or nondiagnostic noninvasive tests
- Pre-operative evaluation for select patients undergoing noncardiac surgery
- Pre-operative evaluation for select patients undergoing surgery for valvular and congenital heart disease
- Evaluation of heart failure syndromes to exclude significant coronary disease
- Other conditions (hypertrophic obstructive cardiomyopathy, aortic dissection, chest trauma)

Table 4.4 Contraindications for coronary angiography

- Patients who do not desire or who are not candidates for revascularization
- Patients in whom revascularization is unlikely to improve quality/duration of life
- As a screening test for CAD in asymptomatic patients
- Routine angiography within 24 hours of lytic therapy in the absence of ongoing ischemia
- Acute renal failure, marked electrolyte imbalance, or metabolic disarray
- Active bleeding or severe coagulopathy
- Prior cholesterol embolization syndrome or anaphylaxis to contrast
- Active infection or unexplained fever
- Decompensated respiratory status, heart failure, or uncontrolled hypertension
- Changing mental status or inability to cooperate

Risks and potential complications

With almost 50 years of procedural refinement, coronary angiography has become a very safe procedure but it does carry some finite risk. Potential complications are listed in *Table 4.5*. The overall risk of developing any complication is <2%, but many of these consist of nonlife-threatening or easily correctable and temporary conditions. The risk of developing a major complication such as death, myocardial infarction (MI) or disabling stroke is roughly 2–3/1000. An example of a serious complication caused by coronary angiography is shown in **4.4**. In this case, coronary angiography was performed to evaluate a patient with a chest pain syndrome. The first view of the LCA (**4.4A**) reveals normal left main, circumflex, and left anterior descending (LAD) arteries. The patient then developed severe chest pain and hypotension and was found to have severe luminal narrowing of the LCA (**4.4B**). This was caused by catheter-induced trauma with an intimal dissection. Fortunately, this complication was successfully treated with a stent. Although this complication is rare and was successfully treated, it may have led to a fatal outcome

Table 4.5 Complications of coronary angiography

- Arrhythmia
- Coronary artery dissection or embolization
- Myocardial infarction
- Heart failure
- Death
- Stroke
- Contrast toxicity/reaction:
  - hypotension and myocardial depression
  - ST/T wave changes
  - allergic reaction (urticaria, bronchospasm, angioedema, laryngospasm, anaphylaxis)
- Renal failure
- Vascular complications:
  - hematoma, AV fistula, pseudo-aneurysm

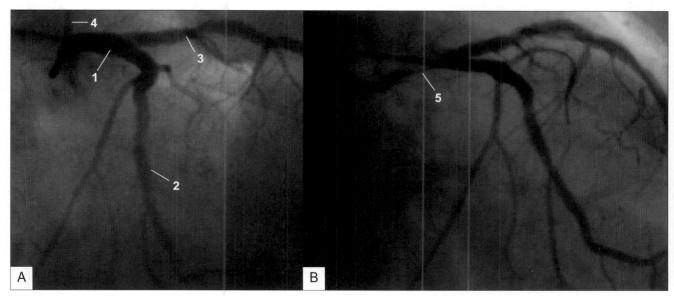

4.4 Coronary angiogram complicated by dissection of the LCA due to catheter trauma. Angiography was performed in a 65-year-old female with chest pain. The left main segment appeared normal without atherosclerotic disease (**A**). On subsequent images it became apparent that the catheter had created a small intimal tear in the left main artery, resulting in a dissection flap leading to luminal compromise of the left main coronary artery (**B**). At this point the patient began to complain of chest pain and became hypotensive. Stent placement in the left main coronary corrected the dissection without further complication. (1: left main stem; 2: left circumflex; 3: left anterior descending; 4: catheter; 5: dissection of left main stem.)

or need for emergency bypass surgery, emphasizing the point that coronary angiography is an invasive procedure that should be performed only in patients with clear indications.

The ionic contrast agents such as diatrizoate meglumine which were commonly used in the earlier days of coronary angiography were notorious for complications such as arrhythmia, hypotension, and myocardial depression and for patient side-effects such as nausea and vomiting. The widespread incorporation of newer, nonionic and isosmolar contrast agents such as iohexol and iodixanol have led to a reduction in these complications and much greater patient comfort, albeit at greater cost. Allergic reactions and renal failure, however, remain important issues. Allergic reactions are typically 'anaphylactoid' (i.e. not IgE-mediated) and typically manifest as urticaria or bronchospasm. More significant manifestations such as respiratory failure and cardiovascular collapse are rare. Patients with known prior contrast reaction can reduce the risk of a contrast reaction by steroid pre-treatment 12 hours prior to contrast administration. Patients at risk for renal toxic effects of contrast include patients with diabetes, pre-existing renal insufficiency, and a dehydrated state. While numerous pharmacologic agents have been tried to prevent contrast-induced nephropathy, simple techniques such as saline hydration, use of nonionic contrast agents, and limiting the dose of contrast are most effective. The use of N-acetylcysteine and sodium bicarbonate is also popular and inexpensive with some apparent benefit.

Limitations

There are numerous limitations of coronary angiography summarized in *Table 4.6*. It is important to emphasize that coronary angiography reveals only the lumen of the artery. A significant amount of coronary disease may be present within the wall of the artery before it encroaches on the lumen and is apparent on angiography. In fact, during the development of atherosclerosis, there is compensatory enlargement of the artery (also known as the 'Glagov phenomenon'), which maintains the lumen despite significant atherosclerosis within the arterial wall[2]. An example of this is shown in **4.5**, where ultrasound images demonstrate a significant amount of plaque in a segment that appeared 'normal' by angiography. Thus, early stages of atherosclerosis escape detection by angiography and disease is not apparent by angiography until there is already a relatively large plaque burden. Furthermore, determination of the severity of a coronary lesion by angiography is dependent on the assumption that there is a normal, nondiseased reference segment with which to compare it. If there is diffuse disease, there is no normal 'reference' segment and thus, angiography will likely underestimate disease severity. Atherosclerosis may lead to eccentric lesions which may have quite complex lumens which, when viewed on angiography, appear as wide as the neighboring segments even in orthogonal views despite causing significant luminal compromise. While eccentric lesions may provide subtle clues to the angiographer such as less

Table 4.6 Limitations of angiography

- Invasive
- Only assesses the lumen; no information on the vessel wall
- Potential underestimation of stenosis severity (diffuse disease, compensatory enlargement of artery, eccentric plaque)
- Ability of angiogram to assess a lesion dependent on quality of image, which is affected by injection technique, body habitus, and lesion and artery characteristics
- Wide interobserver variability/accuracy
- Anatomical information only; no information regarding physiologic significance of lesion

dense opacification or a hazy appearance, such lesions are often not appreciated on angiography.

Importantly, the ability to assess a lesion accurately by angiography is critically dependent on the quality of the image and the ability to visualize the lesion. Numerous technical factors such as catheter size and injection technique greatly affect the quality of the angiogram and the ability to assess a lesion. Body habitus is also very important, with obesity causing poor image quality. Marked vessel tortuosity and the presence of overlapping branches and segments may obscure angiographic findings. These factors have led to the wide interobserver variability well known in coronary angiography. Finally, angiography provides only anatomic information and provides no information on the physiologic effect of a stenosis. This is an important issue in patients with coronary stenoses of moderate severity as it may be unclear if the lesion is flow limiting.

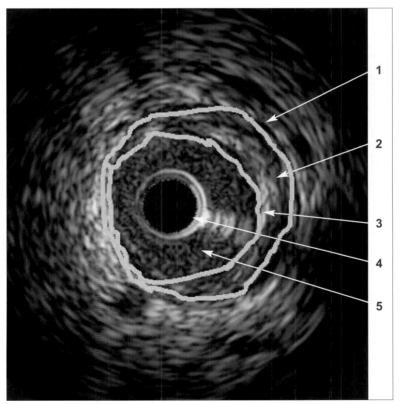

4.5 Intravascular ultrasound image of an arterial segment in the LAD that appeared normal by angiography but demonstrated significant plaque within the arterial wall by intravascular ultrasound. (1: external elastic lamina; 2: plaque in wall of artery; 3: internal elastic lamina; 4: intravascular ultrasound catheter; 5: arterial lumen.)

Similarly, **4.8A** shows a representative view of the LCA from a 55-year-old morbidly obese woman with dyspnea on exertion and a stress perfusion image showing either an anterior reversible defect or breast attenuation artifact. The LCA showed complex anatomy with multiple branches and a segment in the LAD with moderate narrowing that was very difficult to image due to the branches as well as her body habitus. FFR of the LAD was measured and found to be 0.94, indicating that there is no hemodynamic impairment to flow (**4.8B**). Thus, her symptoms likely have a noncoronary explanation.

Intravascular ultrasound (**4.5**) is a clinically useful, invasive adjunct to coronary angiography. The indications for intravascular ultrasound are shown in *Table 4.8*. It can provide careful measurements of the lumen diameter and is the only readily available technique with the ability to image the arterial wall and provide information on plaque characteristics such as the content of lipid, fibrous, and calcific components. Clinically, its main use is as an adjunct to angiography during the performance of coronary interventions and it has proven very helpful in studies of atherosclerosis progression and regression.

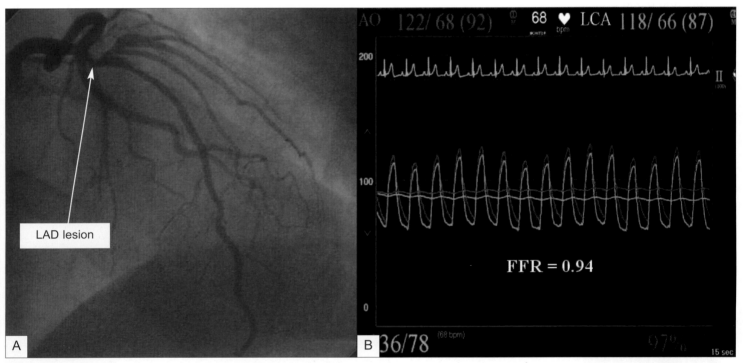

4.8 FFR is helpful to determine the significance of lesions that are not well seen by angiography, due to vessel tortuosity or overlap. A 55-year-old morbidly obese female presented with dyspnea on exertion and a stress perfusion image showing either an anterior reversible defect or breast attenuation artifact. **A**: Angiography of the LCA. A complex moderate narrowing of the proximal LAD is shown (arrow), with multiple branches from the segment making it difficult to assess the severity of the lesion. **B**: Representative waveforms of the adenosine-induced hyperemic pressure gradient, with FFR of 0.94 (not significant).

Table 4.8 Indications for intravascular ultrasound

- Assessment of lesions of moderate severity on angiography
- Accurately measures luminal diameter
- Provides information regarding plaque characteristics:
  - Lipid content
  - Fibrous components
  - Calcification
- Measures plaque volume in progression/regression studies
- Assesses results of intervention:
  - Stent apposition
  - Stent expansion

Clinical scenarios

Patients with angina pectoris often have focal lesions that are amenable to percutaneous intervention. However, coronary disease may be a diffuse process with luminal narrowing affecting a long segment of the coronary artery. When coronary disease is obstructive and diffuse in nature, percutaneous and surgical revascularization options may not be possible or successful at improving symptoms (**4.9**). Chronic total coronary occlusion is a common angiographic finding in patients with angina pectoris. While it is difficult to determine the precise age of an occlusion, several features imply chronicity. These include the absence of a tapering entry point and the presence of 'bridging collaterals'. Bridging collaterals represent dilated vaso vasorum and are small vessels which span the occluded segment, reconstituting flow distal to the occlusion (**4.10**). A total

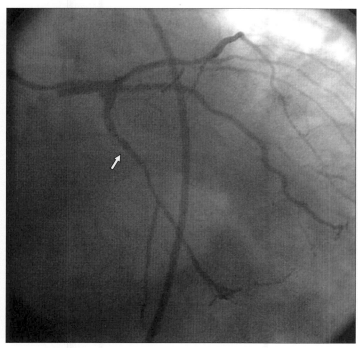

4.9 Example of a diffusely diseased segment of the left circumflex artery (arrow). The small caliber of the vessel and the diffuse nature of the diseased segment would be a challenge for percutaneous or surgical revascularization strategies. This patient's angina was successfully treated with medical therapy.

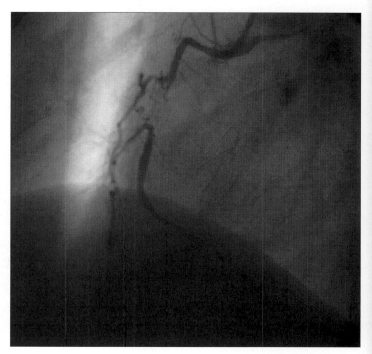

4.10 Example of well-developed, bridging collaterals in a patient with chronic stable angina and total occlusion in the mid-portion of the RCA, with reconstitution of the distal RCA by these collaterals.

occlusion can undergo spontaneous recanalization as illustrated in **4.11**.

Patients with angina may progress to develop an ACS or a STEMI. The underlying pathophysiology is plaque erosion or plaque rupture in the vast majority of cases, being partially/transiently occlusive in ACS and occlusive in STEMI. Coronary angiography performed in this setting may show a highly stenotic lesion with a filling defect distal to the lesion consistent with a thrombus (**4.12**). A variety of coronary angiographic findings may be seen in patients with

ACS. These include the spectrum of a residual noncritical stenosis (**4.13**) to highly obstructive critical left main-stem disease (**4.14**). In the setting of an acute STEMI, the flow pattern in the epicardial coronary artery by angiography is often described using the TIMI perfusion score, based on the early Thrombolysis In Acute Myocardial Infarction Trials. This scale is summarized in *Table 4.9* and describes the contrast flow pattern in the infarct-related coronary artery. The preferred initial treatment of STEMI is mechanical reperfusion, and an example is illustrated in **4.15**.

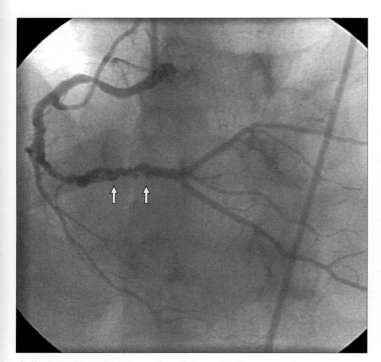

4.11 Arteries with chronic total occlusions can be recanalized, as in this patient with a known totally occluded artery. A recanalized chronic occlusion typically is evident by a 'double lumen' (arrows) representing the recanalized channel.

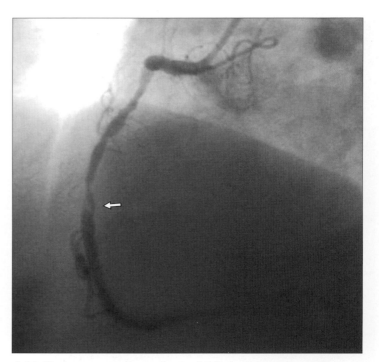

4.12 Coronary angiography in ACS. In this case, a 69-year-old male with several risk factors for CAD presented with prolonged chest pain and ST segment depression which resolved with the initiation of nitrates, beta-blocker, and low molecular weight heparin. Coronary angiography performed the next day showed a highly stenotic lesion in the mid portion of the RCA with a filling defect distal to the lesion consistent with a thrombus (arrow). This lesion was treated successfully with a stent and the use of intravenous adjunctive IIb/IIIa inhibitor.

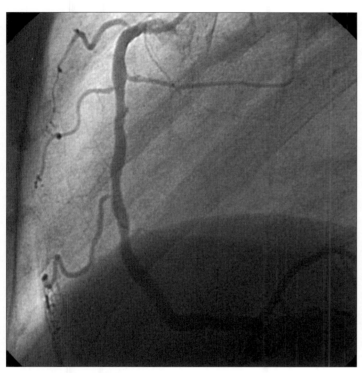

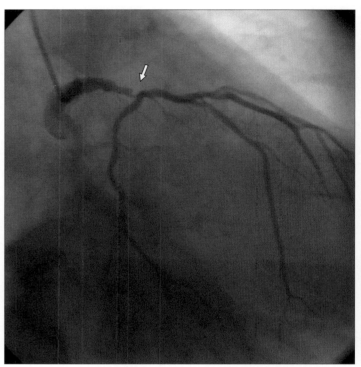

4.13 This representative angiogram of the RCA was obtained in a 41-year-old male smoker presenting with a large, acute inferior wall STEMI. The patient was treated within the first hour with thrombolytic therapy with prompt reperfusion as evidenced by ST segment resolution and improvement in chest pain. This angiogram was obtained 2 days after presentation. There is moderate atherosclerotic narrowing of the RCA without evidence of significant obstruction. The LCA was normal. This case likely represents an example of rupture of a vulnerable but nonobstructing plaque with acute occlusion due primarily to thrombus. Thrombolysis followed by anti-thrombin therapy resolved the thrombus leading to the angiographic findings shown here.

4.14 Left main coronary disease is a potentially life-threatening condition leading to angina pectoris. Coronary angiography can easily identify this important condition. In the example shown here, a patient presenting with stable angina had a 'high-risk' stress test manifested by angina at a low workload, marked ST segment depression early in the exercise portion of the test, and a hypotensive response to exercise. Angiography showed severe narrowing of the distal left main coronary artery (arrow). This patient was referred for coronary bypass surgery.

Table 4.9 The Thrombolysis In Acute Myocardial Infarction Trials (TIMI) scale for grading flow

TIMI score	Flow pattern
0	No contrast past the site of occlusion
1	Small amount of contrast past the site of the occlusion but does not fill the distal vessel
2	Contrast penetrates the site of the occlusion and fills the distal vessel but the rate of filling and washout is slower than that of the noninfarct-related artery
3	Flow beyond the site of occlusion is brisk and normal with a normal rate of contrast washout

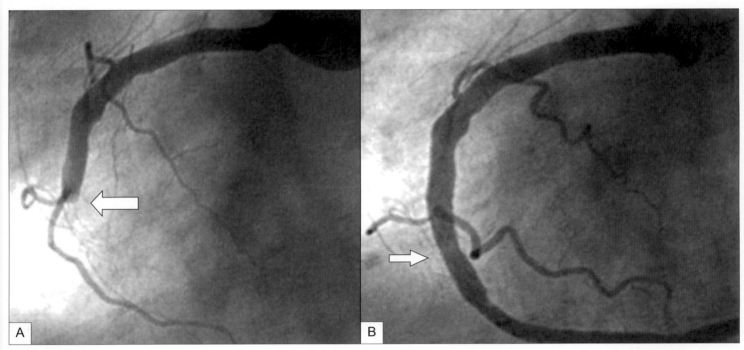

4.15 STEMI is typically due to acute coronary occlusion. Immediate coronary angiography can identify the site of the coronary occlusion and guide revascularization therapy. In this case, a patient with an acute inferior wall STEMI was urgently referred to the cardiac catheterization laboratory. The LCA was normal and, as expected, there is abrupt occlusion of the RCA, representing TIMI 0 flow (**A**). The artery was successfully treated with balloon angioplasty followed by placement of a stent with restoration of normal, TIMI 3 flow in the artery (**B**).

References

1 Scanlon PJ, Faxon DP, Audet AM, *et al.* ACC/AHA guidelines for coronary angiography: a report of the American College of Cardiology/American Heart Association Task Force on Practice Guidelines (Committee on Coronary Angiography). *J Am Coll Cardiol* 1999;**33**:1756–1824.

2 Glagov S, Weisenberg E, Zarins CK, Stankunavicius R, Kolettis GJ. Compensatory enlargement of human atherosclerotic coronary arteries. *NEJM* 1987;**316**:1371–1375.

3 Pijls NH, De Bruyne B, Peels K, *et al.* Measurement of fractional flow reserve to assess the functional severity of coronary artery stenoses. *NEJM* 1996;**334**:1703–1708.

Further reading

Aude YW, Garza L. How to prevent unnecessary coronary interventions: identifying lesions responsible for ischemia in the cath lab. *Curr Opin Cardiol* 2003;**18**:394–399.

Bishop AH, Samady H. Fractional flow reserve: critical review of an important physiology adjunct to angiography. *Am Heart J* 2004;**147**:792–802.

Guedes A, Tardiff JC. Intravascular ultrasound assessment of atherosclerosis. *Curr Atheroscler Rep* 2004;**6**:219–224.

Kern MJ, de Bruyne B, Pijls NH. From research to clinical practice: current role of intracoronary physiologically based decision making in the cardiac catheterization laboratory. *J Am Coll Cardiol* 1997;**30**:613–620.

Chapter 5

Nonatherosclerotic causes of angina pectoris and ischemia

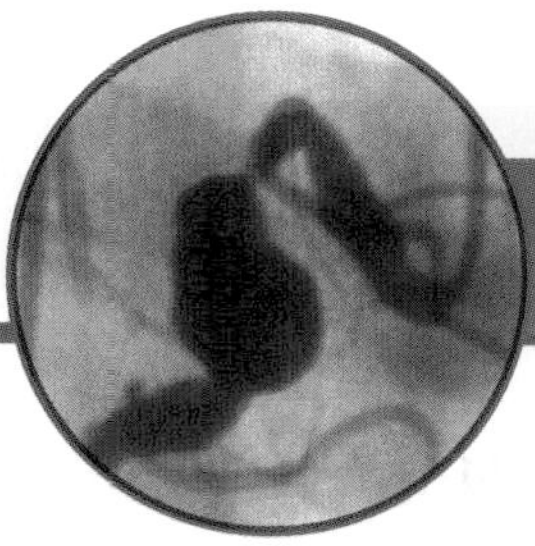

Michael Ragosta, MD

Introduction

Coronary artery disease (CAD) resulting in significant luminal narrowing is responsible for most cases of angina pectoris. There are, however, other causes of angina pectoris and myocardial ischemia that are not due to atherosclerotic narrowing of the coronary artery. Coronary angiography is often necessary to define the underlying etiology. It is helpful to classify these conditions into those that are associated with arterial obstruction from conditions other than atherosclerotic narrowing and thus associated with diminished supply to the myocardium, versus conditions in which the coronary arteries are without obstruction yet are unable to meet the increased myocardial demand for blood. The nonatherosclerotic causes of angina pectoris and myocardial ischemia are outlined in *Table 5.1*.

Table 5.1 Nonatherosclerotic causes of angina pectoris

Nonatherosclerotic obstruction
- Coronary artery spasm
- Microcirculation abnormalities
- Coronary anomalies
- Myocardial bridging
- Coronary embolism
- Coronary dissection

Nonobstructive coronaries
- Ventricular hypertrophy
- Anemia, hypoxemia
- Thyrotoxicosis
- Tachycardia, hypertensive crisis

anomaly. Similarly, the anomalous left circumflex originating from the RCA or right coronary cusp is one of the most common anomalies observed (**5.2**). However, several specific coronary anomalies are associated with angina and sudden cardiac death. These include: (1) the anomalous origin of the LCA from the right sinus of Valsalva coursing between the pulmonary artery and the aorta; (2) a single coronary artery usually arising from the right aortic sinus, and (3) anomalous origin of the LCA

from the pulmonary trunk. Rarely, coronary anomalies may lead to ischemia. The mechanism by which coronary anomalies cause myocardial ischemia is not clearly established. It is thought that angina is observed in these rare entities from compression of the coronary artery by the great vessels during exertion, or from the acute angulation of the proximal segment of the anomalous vessel which is necessary to reach its ultimate vascular territory (*Table 5.4*).

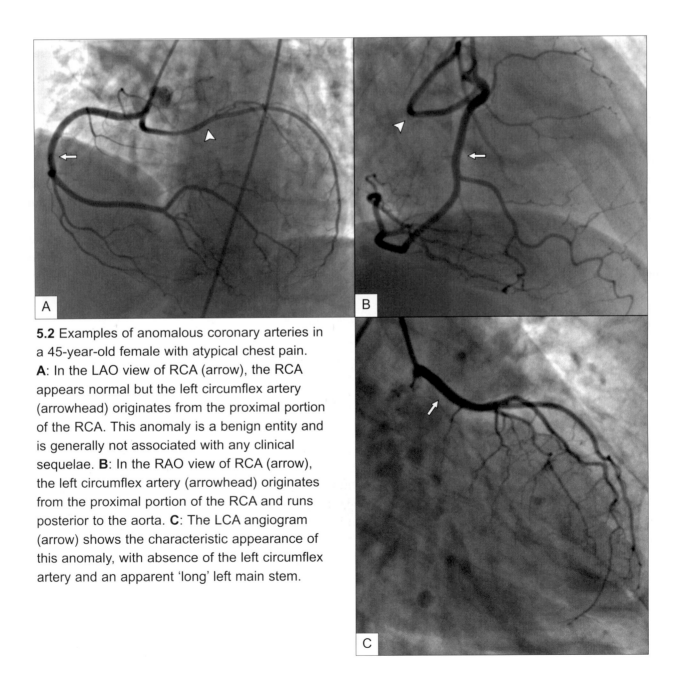

5.2 Examples of anomalous coronary arteries in a 45-year-old female with atypical chest pain.
A: In the LAO view of RCA (arrow), the RCA appears normal but the left circumflex artery (arrowhead) originates from the proximal portion of the RCA. This anomaly is a benign entity and is generally not associated with any clinical sequelae. **B**: In the RAO view of RCA (arrow), the left circumflex artery (arrowhead) originates from the proximal portion of the RCA and runs posterior to the aorta. **C**: The LCA angiogram (arrow) shows the characteristic appearance of this anomaly, with absence of the left circumflex artery and an apparent 'long' left main stem.

Table 5.4 Mechanisms of ischemia from coronary anomalies

- Shunting and coronary steal
- Acute angulation of the aortocoronary junction
- 'Slit-like' ostium
- Compression between the great vessels

Table 5.5 Potential sources of coronary embolism

- Left atrium/appendage
- Left ventricular thrombus
- Prosthetic valve thrombus
- Aortic valve endocarditis
- Mitral valve endocarditis
- Coronary artery aneurysm

Myocardial bridges represent an intramyocardial segment of a coronary artery. This condition typically involves the mid-portion of the left anterior descending artery (LAD) and is observed on angiography as systolic compression of the coronary artery (**5.3**). It remains debatable whether myocardial bridges lead to significant ischemia and it is generally agreed that a myocardial bridge is an uncommon cause of angina pectoris. Nevertheless, there are many examples of patients with anginal syndromes who are subsequently found to have a myocardial bridge on coronary angiography, and improve with stenting or revascularization of the involved segment.

Coronary embolism may rarely result in an acute anginal syndrome. There are several potential sources of coronary embolism (*Table 5.5*). The most common source is the left atrium and left atrial appendage in the setting of atrial fibrillation. The left ventricle may also be a source of embolism, particularly from mural thrombus after large anterior wall myocardial infarctions (MIs) or severe left ventricular dysfunction. Coronary emboli may also originate

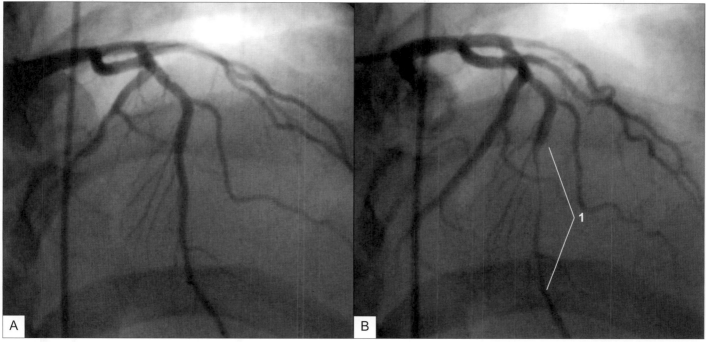

5.3 Left coronary angiograms in a 40-year-old male with an atypical anginal syndrome, demonstrating a myocardial bridge. Catheterization showed a normal RCA. **A**: During diastole, the mid-portion of the LAD appears normal. **B**: During systole, this segment becomes markedly narrowed with near obliteration, consistent with a myocardial bridge (1).

from an infected mitral or aortic valve (**5.4**) or from thrombosis of an aortic or mitral prosthetic valve. Coronary artery aneurysms are another potential, albeit rare, source of coronary embolism (**5.5**). The most common cause of a coronary aneurysm is atherosclerotic coronary disease but aneurysms may also occur as sequelae of Kawasaki's disease. The optimal treatment for this condition is not well known; many clinicians would treat such patients with warfarin and/or anti-platelet agents. Frequently, smaller aneurysms are found in association with other atherosclerotic coronary disease and are clinically unimportant.

Dissection of the coronary artery can occur in association with acute aortic dissection involving the ascending arch of the aorta, and can lead to acute onset of anginal chest pain. Coronary artery dissection can rarely occur spontaneously. This rare entity has been described in patients with Ehlers–Danlos syndrome and in post-partum females (**5.6**). Occasionally, coronary spasm may be observed in the cardiac catheterization laboratory as an artifact from catheter positioning (**5.7**). This does not imply that the individual has vasospastic angina.

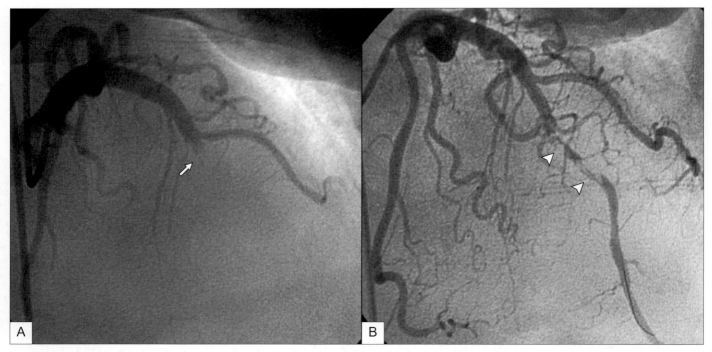

5.4 A: An example of a coronary embolism from endocarditis of the aortic valve in a 70-year-old female with hypertension who presented with acute onset of chest pain and shortness of breath; the EKG demonstrated an acute anterior STEMI. On catheterization total occlusion was noted in the mid-portion of the LAD (arrow). The remainder of her coronary arteries were normal with no evidence of atherosclerosis. **B**: After balloon angioplasty, there were clear filling defects in the vessel as demonstrated (arrowheads), which did not respond to anti-thrombotic therapy. Echocardiography performed post-procedure demonstrated active endocarditis of the aortic valve with vegetations. Given the behavior of the lesion, the lack of coronary disease elsewhere and the presence of active endocarditis with valvular vegetations, the coronary likely was occluded from embolism of an infected vegetation due to endocarditis.

5.5 Multiple large RCA aneurysms (arrows) in a 72-year-old male with multiple coronary risk factors (hypertension, dyslipidemia, tobacco abuse) and presentation with prolonged rest pain and inferior changes on his EKG with positive serum biomarkers consistent with a STEMI. Several large aneurysmal segments of the RCA were noted without evidence of luminal narrowing elsewhere in the artery. There was no significant disease in the LCA, although several segments of the LAD were ectactic but not aneurysmal. Based on the clinical history and the angiograms, it was concluded that the RCA aneurysm led to development of thrombus with distal embolization, leading to an acute ischemic syndrome.

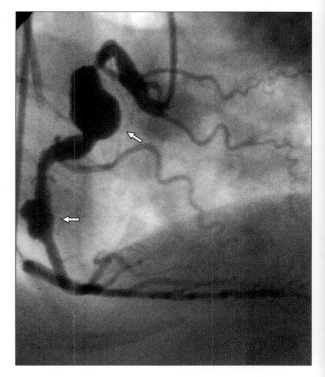

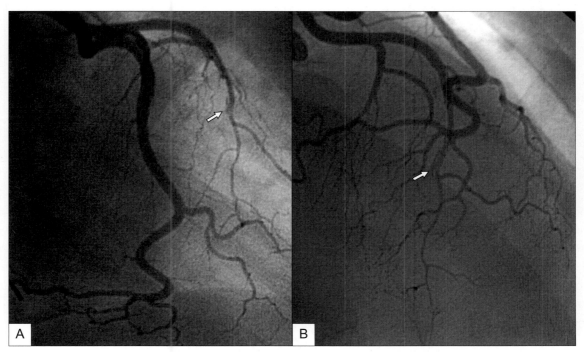

5.6 Example of a spontaneous dissection of the LAD resulting in an acute ischemic syndrome. The coronary arteries appear normal except for the LAD, which demonstrated a long narrowing (arrows), beginning in the mid-portion of the vessel and extending to the apical portion. A small, linear extravasation of contrast can be seen at the tip of the arrows, consistent with the site of the spontaneous coronary dissection. **A:** RAO caudal view. **B:** RAO cranial view.

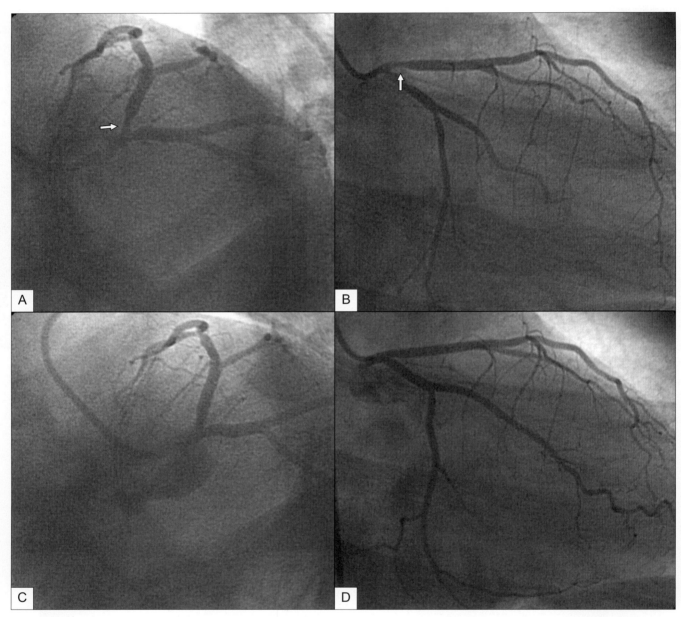

5.7 Angiograms from a 46-year-old female with several risk factors for CAD and atypical chest pain with a normal EKG during chest pain and no biomarker evidence of ischemia. The RCA angiogram was normal. **A**: LCA in the LAO caudal view demonstrating a stenosis in the LAD at the tip of the diagnostic catheter (arrow). **B**: LCA in the RAO caudal view demonstrating LAD stenosis (arrow). **C,D**: Following sublingual nitroglycerin, the apparent stenosis resolved. Differentiation of catheter-induced spasm from an atherosclerotic stenosis is critical for the correct management of this patient.

Nonobstructive causes of angina

There are several common conditions which lead to angina pectoris in the absence of coronary artery obstruction because of increased myocardial oxygen consumption. In such cases, the coronary arteries appear normal but the supply is inadequate to meet the increased demand. The most common such condition is severe left ventricular hypertrophy, which may be due to long-standing hypertension, aortic stenosis, or hypertrophic cardiomyopathy. In addition to the increased muscle mass leading to increased wall tension and myocardial oxygen demand, patients with left ventricular hypertrophy also have abnormalities of the microcirculation leading to impaired coronary flow reserve.

Severe anemia and hypoxemia can cause angina in the absence of epicardial coronary obstruction from diminished oxygen supply in the face of normal or increased demand. Finally, any condition leading to tachycardia or marked hypertension can lead to increased myocardial oxygen demand and angina in the setting of normal coronaries. Such conditions include fever, thyrotoxicosis, tachycardia from a variety of arrhythmias, and hypertensive urgency or crisis. Any of these conditions may mimic the acute ischemic syndromes and, in fact, there may be release of biomarkers such as troponin with severe episodes. However, it is very important to diagnose these conditions properly since the management approach differs entirely from true acute ischemic syndromes, which are due to plaque rupture and thrombus formation.

Further reading

Angeline P. Normal and anomalous coronary arteries: definitions and classification. *Am Heart J* 1989;**117**:418–434.

Basso C, Maron BJ, Corrado D, Thiene G. Clinical profile of congenital artery anomalies with origin from the wrong aortic sinus leading to sudden death in young competitive athletes. *J Am Coll Cardiol* 2000;**35**:1493–1501.

Crea F, Lanza GA. Angina pectoris and normal coronary arteries: cardiac syndrome X. *Heart* 2004;**90**:457–463.

Kashki JC, Aldama G, Cosin-Sales J. Cardiac syndrome X. Diagnosis, pathogenesis, and management. *Am J Cardiovasc Drugs* 2004;**4**:179–194.

Konidala S, Gutterman DD. Coronary vasospasm and the regulation of coronary blood flow. *Prog Cardiovasc Dis* 2004;**46**:349–373.

Mayer S, Hillis LD. Prinzmetal's variant angina. *Clin Cardiol* 1998;**21**:243–246.

Kawano H, Ogawa H. Endothelial function and coronary spastic angina. *Intern Med* 2005;**44**:91–99.

Mirza MA. Angina-like pain and normal coronary arteries. Uncovering cardiac syndromes that mimic CAD. *Postgrad Med* 2005;**117**:41–46.

Rapp AH, Hillis LD. Clinical consequences of anomalous coronary arteries. *Coron Artery Dis* 2001;**12**:617–620.

Chapter 6

An approach to the management of chronic angina

Ian J Sarembock, MB, ChB, MD

Introduction

Although definitive data on the incidence and prevalence of chronic stable angina (CSA) are sparse, the worldwide demographic tide of an aging population and the explosive increase in the incidence of type 2 diabetes mellitus will almost certainly result in a rapid acceleration in the rate of coronary artery disease (CAD) and angina in the next decade. World Health Organization (WHO) projections suggest that in 2020 CAD will remain a major cause for concern, accounting for 5.9% of the total global disease burden and 11.2% of that in developed regions[1]. CSA is the initial manifestation of CAD in approximately half of all presenting patients. It is important not only because of its prevalence but also because of its associated morbidity and mortality. In the United States, the annual rate of myocardial infarction (MI) in patients with symptoms of angina is 3.0–3.5% (i.e. 1 million patients) but, more importantly, approximately half of this group suffer sudden cardiac death before reaching the hospital[2]. Many more are hospitalized for unstable angina and evaluation and treatment of stable chest pain syndromes. Others have debilitating chronic chest pain syndromes collectively reflected by a considerable economic burden of stable angina, which contributes to annual Medicare payments in the region of $7.5 billion and total hospitalization costs (including non-Medicare patients) of approximately twice this amount.

The current American College of Cardiology/American Heart Association (ACC/AHA) guidelines for the management of CSA focus on both risk assessment and treatment in symptomatic as well as asymptomatic patients with known or suspected CAD[2]. The goals of therapy of CSA are: (1) amelioration of anginal symptoms and

improved angina-free exertion capability, and (2) prevention or reduction of subsequent acute MI, unstable angina (UA), or ischemic sudden death (ISD).

In asymptomatic patients, risk stratification and prognosis are more important considerations than diagnosis. In this group there are clear advantages of treating high-risk patients, because the aim must be to protect against MI and prolong life. Moreover, prevention of risk factors for CAD also reduces the risk of stroke. The most important step in evaluating symptomatic patients with chest pain is the clinical examination, including a thorough history and physical examination. This 'low tech' approach allows the clinician to estimate with a high degree of accuracy the likelihood of clinically significant CAD[3]. Clinico-pathologic studies have confirmed that the simple clinical observations of pain type, age, and gender are powerful predictors of the likelihood of CAD[4]. Based on these parameters, a 52-year-old obese, sedentary male with typical angina has a 94% likelihood of having significant CAD, whereas a 35-year-old anxious female without defined risk factors and atypical effort chest pain has a 1% chance of developing CAD. A number of co-existing vascular risk factors including hyperlipidemia, diabetes mellitus, systemic hypertension, smoking, or known vascular disease (including MI, history of revascularization, stroke, transient ischemic attack, or peripheral vascular disease) are strong predictors of CAD and significantly elevate the risk[5,6]. It is recommended by the AHA that evaluations using resting 12-lead electrocardiograms (EKGs), although less predictive than medical history, should also be recorded in all patients with symptoms suggestive of angina pectoris[2]. However, an abnormal EKG will be found in no more than 50% of

concluded that guideline-compliant medical therapy

6.2). The importance of treating high blood pressure in

Table 6.2 Treatment of stable angina pectoris

Patient characteristics	Treatment
All patients	Daily aspirin Smoking cessation Treat dyslipidemia Control of high blood pressure to levels ≤140/90 mmHg (to 130/80 mmHg in diabetes mellitus)
Left main to three-vessel coronary artery disease with decreased left ventricular function	CABG surgery (if feasible) ACE inhibitor and β-blockers when ejection fraction <40%
One-, two-, or three-vessel disease with normal left ventricular function	Anti-anginal drug treatment Percutaneous transluminal coronary angioplasty or CABG surgery if symptoms are not controlled with drug treatment
Refractory angina, very poor left ventricular function or not a candidate for revascularization	Consider bepridil, external enhanced counterpulsation, transmyocardial laser revascularization, spinal cord stimulation, trans-thoracic sympathetic denervation or heart transplant

(Adapted from Crawford MH, DiMarco JP, Paulus WJ (eds). *Cardiology*, 2nd edn. Elsevier, Oxford, 2004.)

patients with CSA, and ambulatory EKG findings during chest pain are abnormal only in about half of patients with angina who have a normal resting EKG.

Exercise testing is a well-established and widely used diagnostic tool that is generally safe, yet both MI and death occur at a rate of approximately 1 per 2,500 tests[7]. Furthermore, a meta-analysis of 147 published reports describing 24,074 patients who underwent both coronary angiography and exercise testing found wide variation in its sensitivity and specificity[8]. Although stress imaging procedures (either stress myocardial perfusion imaging or stress echocardiography) are commonly used in symptomatic patients and increase the sensitivity and specificity of exercise EKG testing, it is only indicated as an initial test in asymptomatic patients with resting EKG abnormalities that preclude adequate interpretation of the exercise EKG. These include patients with pre-excitation or baseline nonspecific ST depression. Pharmacologic stress imaging is considered preferable to exercise EKG testing for patients who are unable to exercise.

Resting systolic pump function as measured by left

suggest that high levels of newer biomarkers including high-sensitivity C-reactive protein or brain natriuretic peptide indicate a poor prognosis, at present, routine measurement is not recommended.

Goals of therapy

The primary objectives of therapy for chronic stable angina are: (1) to provide symptomatic relief by limiting or eliminating angina, thus allowing the patient to return to normal daily activities, and (2) to prevent disease progression and its sequelae, including a reduction in mortality and morbidity (*Table 6.1*). Ideally these goals should be successfully accomplished with the minimum of side-effects. Many of the recommended medications have unfavorable side-effects, including impotence, fatigue, edema, and severe headaches. Although not life threatening, the side-effects of medical treatment affect quality of life and, in so doing, prevent patients from carrying out normal daily activities. Treatment of side-effects, especially those

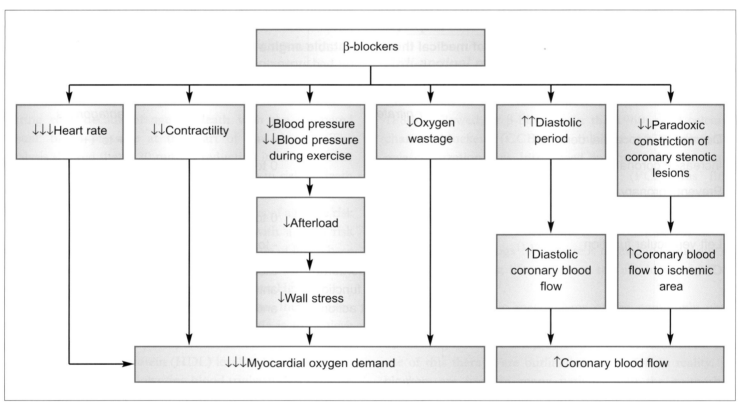

6.2 Mechanisms of action of β-blockers. (Adapted from Crawford MH, DiMarco JP, Paulus WJ (eds). *Cardiology*, 2nd edn. Elsevier, Oxford, 2004.)

Table 6.5 Adverse effects of beta-adrenergic blocking agents

Cardiac
- Increased ventricular volume resulting in congestive heart failure
- Excessive heart rate slowing or heart block
- Withdrawal syndrome

Noncardiac
- Fatigue
- Mental depression
- Insomnia
- Hallucinations
- Bad dreams
- Gastrointestinal upset
- Sexual dysfunction

- Raynaud's phenomenon
- Worsened claudication symptoms
- Bronchoconstriction
- Further renal deterioration in patients with renal disease

Metabolic
- Increased LDL cholesterol and triglycerides; lowered HDL cholesterol
- Worsening of insulin-induced hypoglycemia; masking of hypoglycemic symptoms
- Increased blood sugar in insulin-resistant diabetics

oxygen demand. By improving diastolic blood flow, they increase blood flow to ischemic myocardium, which in turn results in an overall improvement in coronary blood flow. The side-effects of β-blocker therapy can be troublesome (*Table 6.5*). These are grouped into cardiac, noncardiac, and metabolic. Although the list of side-effects is lengthy, the overall benefits of these agents far outweigh the side-effects and thus they remain the primary therapy for patients with chronic angina.

An alternative to a β-blocker would be a CCB (*Tables 6.6, 6.7*, **6.3**, **6.4**). Although CCBs increase heart rate, they also result in decreased contractility and vasodilatation, which

---

Table 6.6 Candidates for calcium channel blocking agent therapy

Ideal candidates
- With co-existent hypertension
- Believed to have episodes of vasoconstriction (mixed angina) or vasospasm
- With supraventricular arrhythmia (verapamil or diltiazem)

Poor candidates
- Severe left ventricular dysfunction or congestive heart failure
- Bradyarrhythmias (sinus bradycardia, slow atrial fibrillation, atrioventricular node block); such individuals should not be given verapamil or diltiazem

---

Table 6.7 Adverse effects of calcium channel blocking agents

Symptom	Cause	Implicated calcium channel antagonist
Dizziness, light-headedness, syncope, palpitation	Excessive hypotension Bradycardia Reflex tachycardia	All Verapamil, diltiazem Dihydropyridines
Exacerbation or precipitation of congestive heart failure	Negative inotropic action	Most; amlodipine, felodipine are the safest to use, even in heart failure
Severe bradycardia or heart block	Negative chronotropic action; especially sick sinus node disease	Verapamil, diltiazem
Precipitation of angina	Hypotension, coronary steal	Nifedipine and possibly other dihydropyridines

---

Oral	20–30 mg	Twice daily given 7–8 hours apart
Oral sustained release	60–240 mg	Once daily

*Very limited data available on efficacy

Dihydropyridine calcium channel blockers

Table 6.10 Adverse effects of long-acting nitrates

Effect	Occurrence
Headache	Common
Nausea and vomiting	Occasional
Dizziness or overt syncope	Occasional
Palpitations and tachycardia	Uncommon
Tolerance and attenuation	Common

Table 6.11 Mechanisms of clinical tolerance to long-acting nitrates

- Decreased availability of intracellular sulfhydryl groups involved in the conversion of the parent organic nitrate to nitric oxide; this mechanism may involve the enzyme responsible for nitrate bioconversion to nitric oxide
- Neurohormonal activation with increased circulating catecholamines, renin, angiotensin, and vasopressin, which results in enhanced systemic vasoconstrictor activity
- Plasma volume expansion
- Deranged enzymatic conversion of nitrate to nitric oxide

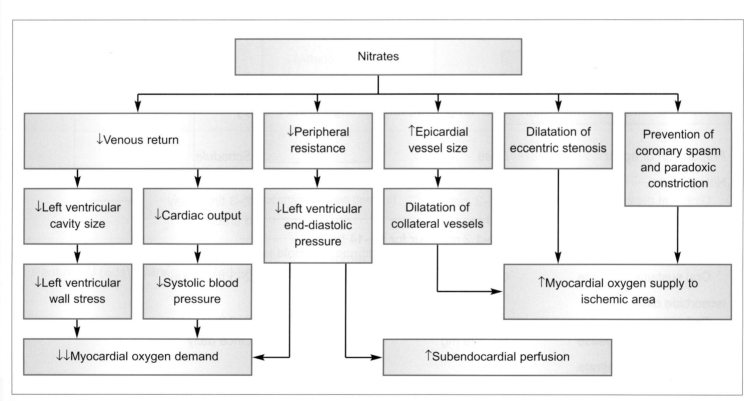

6.5 Mechanism of action of long-acting nitrates. (Adapted from Crawford MH, DiMarco JP, Paulus WJ (eds). *Cardiology*, 2nd edn. Elsevier, Oxford, 2004.)

important so as to prevent nitrate tolerance (*Table 6.11*); continuous therapy produces rapid tolerance. Intermittent therapy, with daily nitrate-free intervals, usually in the order of 10–12 hours, prevents clinical nitrate tolerance (*Table 6.12*)[11].

Optimal tolerated doses of anti-anginal drugs should be used, and often 2 agents are necessary[11]. If the patient does not respond adequately to monotherapy, combination therapy of a β-blocker with a long-acting dihydropyridine CCB or a long-acting nitrate should be tried (*Table 6.13*). However, some combinations are unwise or even dangerous; the combination of β-blocker plus the rate-slowing CCBs verapamil or diltiazem has a high probability of causing atrioventricular block, including complete heart block, especially in the elderly. Therapy with three drugs is often used in clinical practice, but there are few objective data to support the idea that treatment with three drugs is superior to that with two agents[11]. This is often the consequence of side-effects at higher doses of individual agents. It is important to use the maximum dose(s) of anti-anginal agent(s) that the patient can tolerate.

Table 6.12 Avoidance of clinical tolerance to long-acting nitrates

- Use smallest effective dose
- Administer the fewest possible doses per day
- Avoid continuous or sustained exposure to nitrates
- Provide a nitrate-free interval of ±10 hours/day

Coronary artery revascularization

An initial trial of anti-anginal drugs is indicated for the vast majority of patients with stable angina. However, a significant number of patients will continue to have angina despite optimally tolerated medical therapy and, in these cases, revascularization procedures should be considered. This therapeutic option is particularly relevant for those who lead an active lifestyle, for subjects with a large ischemic burden on perfusion imaging, and for those with severe CAD, especially with decreased LV function (*Table 6.14*)[11,13]. Relief of angina after revascularization is greater than with medical therapy (*Table 6.15*). The Angioplasty compared to Medicine (ACME) study sought to assess outcomes of men with double- and single-vessel coronary artery disease randomly assigned to treatment by percutaneous transluminal coronary angioplasty (PTCA) or medical therapy, compared with previously reported outcomes for men with single-vessel disease. Male patients (n = 328) with stable angina pectoris and ischemia on treadmill testing were randomly assigned to PTCA or medical therapy; 101 patients had double-vessel disease, and 227 had single-vessel disease. Symptoms, treadmill performance, quality of life score, coronary stenosis, and myocardial perfusion were compared at baseline and at 6 months. Patients were followed-up for up to 6 years and underwent additional treadmill testing 2–3 years after randomization. PTCA treated and medically treated patients with double-vessel disease experienced comparable improvement in exercise duration (+1.2 *vs.* +1.3 min, respectively, $p = 0.89$), freedom from angina (53% and 36%, respectively, $p = 0.09$) and improvement of overall quality of life score (+1.3 *vs.* +4.4, respectively, $p = 0.32$) at 6 months compared with baseline. This contrasts with greater

Table 6.13 Combinations of anti-anginal therapies

Combination	Beneficial	Should be avoided or is relatively contraindicated
Nitrates + β-blockers	X	
Nitrates + diltiazem, verapamil	X	
Nitrates + dihydropyridine		X
β-blockers + dihydropyridine	X	
β-blockers + diltiazem, verapamil		X

Table 6.14 Factors in selecting mechanical revascularization over medical therapy in angina

Clinical
- Poor or partial response to intensive medical therapy
- Lifestyle (occupation, recreation) limited stable angina on medical therapy

Noninvasive
- Objective evidence for major ischemia
- Strongly positive stress test (low workload, ST-segment depression ≥2 mm, failure of systolic blood pressure to rise, early onset of ischemia)
- Large, reversible thallium defect; two or more reversible thallium defects; increased lung thallium uptake
- Extensive or multiple wall motion abnormalities on stress echocardiography or stress radionuclide angiography
- Strongly positive ambulatory recording: >4 episodes of ST depression/day; >30 minutes of ST depression/day

Invasive
- Main left coronary artery stenosis or three-vessel disease, especially if LV function is decreased (CABG)
- Two-vessel disease with decreased LV function and/or proximal LAD involvement
- Two-vessel disease with frequent symptoms or ischemia on noninvasive testing while on medical therapy
- One-vessel disease with easily induced ischemia on medical therapy (PTCA)

Table 6.15 Efficacy of angioplasty *vs.* medical therapy in single-vessel disease (ACME study)

Outcome	Medical therapy (n = 107) (%)	PTCA (n = 105) (%)	P value
PTCA	10	96	-
rePTCA	9	16	-
CABG	0	7	<0.010
ETT duration	+0.5 minutes	+2.2 minutes	<0.001
Decrease in angina frequency	-7/month	-15/month	0.060
Angina free	46	64	<0.010
Myocardial infarction	3	5	-
Death	1	0	-

advantages favoring PTCA by these criteria in patients with single-vessel disease ($p = 0.0001$ to 0.02). Trends present at 6 months persisted at late follow-up. Patients undergoing double-vessel dilation had less complete initial revascularization (45% *vs.* 83%) and greater average stenosis of worst lesions at 6 months (74% *vs.* 56%). Likewise, patients with double-vessel disease showed less improved myocardial perfusion imaging (59% *vs.* 75%).

The authors concluded that PTCA is beneficial in male patients with double-vessel disease; however, the same advantage over medical therapy was not seen in similar patients with single-vessel disease. Less complete revascularization and greater restenosis for patients having multiple dilations could account for these findings. Technical advances since completion of this trial might improve these outcomes and are indeed the case with the development of stent techniques including the use of drug-eluting stents. In the two- to three-year follow-up of patients with single-vessel coronary artery disease randomized to PTCA versus medical therapy had sustained benefit, making it an attractive therapeutic option for these patients (*Table 6.15*).

Unfortunately, angina often recurs after percutaneous coronary intervention or coronary artery bypass grafting (CABG). As highlighted by the recent ARTS Trial, only 20–40% of patients undergoing either percutaneous or surgical revascularization are free of angina and not requiring adjunctive medical therapy one year after optimal revascularization (*Table 6.16*). In this trial, a total of 1205 patients were randomly assigned to undergo stent implantation or bypass surgery when a cardiac surgeon and an interventional cardiologist agreed that the same extent of revascularization could be achieved by either technique. The primary clinical endpoint was freedom from major adverse cardiac and cerebrovascular events at 1 year. At 1 year, there was no significant difference between the two groups in terms of the rates of death, stroke, or MI. Among patients who survived without a stroke or an MI, 16.8% of those in the stent group underwent a second revascularization, as compared with 3.5% of those in the surgery group. The rate of event-free survival at 1 year was 73.8% among the patients who received stents and 87.8% among those who underwent bypass surgery (*p*<0.001 by the log-rank test). As measured 1 year after the procedure, coronary stenting for multi-vessel disease is less expensive than bypass surgery and offers the same degree of protection against death, stroke, and MI. However, stenting is associated with a greater need for repeated revascularization. In addition, 60–80% of patients are still taking some form of anti-anginal medication and 10–20% are still having angina. Compared with medical therapy, these procedures therefore do not prolong life or reduce the incidence of MI, except in patients with severe left main CAD and in those with 2- or 3-vessel disease with decreased LV function, for whom CABG surgery (in retrospective subgroup analyses of the published data) has demonstrated improved survival[2,11,12]. Results of the efficacy of balloon angioplasty versus CABG on long-term sequelae are summarized in *Table 6.17*. The major difference between these two therapeutic strategies was the need for repeat revascularization. This gap has been significantly narrowed by the use of coronary stents.

Clinical restenosis occurs in 20–30% of patients undergoing percutaneous intervention with bare metal stents; restenosis rates are significantly higher in patients with diabetes mellitus. Restenosis is considerably lower with patients receiving drug-eluting stents (10%), but appears to be higher in patients with diabetes. In addition, late stent thrombosis, occurring 12–24 months after successful stent placement, remains a concern[11]. Following surgical revascularization, venous bypass graft occlusions occur in >50% of grafts by 10 years after surgery. For this reason, arterial conduits are generally preferred and are critically important in patients with diabetes.

Table 6.16 Efficacy of revascularization *vs.* medical therapy on angina (ARTS study)

Variable	12 months after intervention		
	Stenting group (%)	Surgery group (%)	P value
Free of angina	78.9	89.5	<0.001
Free of anti-anginal medication	21.1	41.5	<0.001
Free of angina and anti-anginal medication	19.1	38.4	<0.001

~60–80% are still taking anti-anginal medications
~10–20% still have angina

(Adapted from Serruys PW, *et al.* Comparison of coronary-artery bypass surgery and stenting for the treatment of multivessel disease. *N Engl J Med* 2001;**344**:1117–1124.)

Table 6.17 Efficacy of PTCA *vs.* CABG on long-term sequelae

Trial	Patients (n)	Follow-up (y)	Mortality (%)		Myocardial infarction (%)		Repeat revascularization (%)	
			PTCA	CABG	PTCA	CABG	PTCA	CABG
EAST	392	1.0	7.0	7.0	14.0	19.0	62.0	13.0
RITA	1,101	2.5	3.1	3.6	6.6	5.2	38.0*	11.0
GABI	359	1.0	1.6	2.8	2.7	9.0*	44.0*	6.0
CABRI	1,067	1.0	3.4	3.1	2.9	3.3	34.0*	7.0
ERACI	127	1.0	4.7	4.7	9.5	7.8	36.0*	17.0

EAST (Emory Angioplasty *vs.* Surgery) Trial, *Am J Cardiol* 1997;**79**(11):1453–1459
RITA (Randomized Intervention Trial of unstable Angina) Trial, *Lancet* 1993;**341**:573–580
GABI (German Angioplasty Bypass Surgery Investigation) Trial, *N Engl J Med* 1994;**331**:1037–1043
CABRI (Coronary Angioplasty *vs.* Bypass Revascularization Investigation) Trial, *Lancet* 1995;**346**(8984):1179–1184
ERACI (Argentine Randomized Trial of Percutaneous Transluminal Coronary Angioplasty *vs.* Coronary Artery Bypass Surgery in Multivessel Disease) Trial, *J Am Coll Cardiol* 1993;**22**(4):1060–1067
*$p<0.001$

Strategies to reduce major adverse clinical outcomes

Although anti-anginal drugs and revascularization procedures provide symptomatic relief, they do not reduce the incidence of ISD, MI, or acute coronary syndrome (ACS), which frequently occur in patients with CSA[2, 11–13]. Adverse outcomes occur at random and are typically caused by plaque rupture or erosion[14]. To reduce these undesirable clinical outcomes, vasculo-protective strategies must be used in addition to anti-anginal drugs.

Smoking cessation

Smoking cessation is critically important for all patients with CSA and reduces the risk of coronary artery mortality by up to 50% in 1 year[15]. It also has a positive effect on exercise performance in CSA. Nevertheless, our ability to be successful in achieving this goal is low and in most cases it takes a multi-disciplinary approach and high motivation on the part of the patient.

Aspirin

Daily aspirin is recommended for all patients with CSA, unless there is a specific contraindication, such as aspirin allergy or a history of an upper gastrointestinal (GI) hemorrhage. In a previous report, daily aspirin (325 mg) reduced cardiovascular mortality and morbidity with an absolute reduction of 12 additional deaths for every 1000

patients with CSA treated during a 15-month period[16]. Other data have shown beneficial effects of daily aspirin for patients with acute MI and ACS[11]. Low-dose aspirin (81–100 mg) is generally recommended. Thus, aspirin is an inexpensive and effective way of reducing adverse clinical outcomes in CSA.

Clopidogrel

No outcome studies currently exist with the use of clopidogrel in patients with CSA who have not undergone percutaneous coronary revascularization with stents. Current guidelines recommend the use of clopidogrel as an alternative to aspirin in patients with known allergic reactions to aspirin or upper GI bleeding. However, in a study of patients with a history of upper GI bleeding due to ulcers, the recurrence of bleeding was 12 times greater during clopidogrel treatment compared with treatment with aspirin and a proton pump inhibitor (PPI). Thus, for the present, if cardiac prophylaxis is necessary in patients with a history of an upper GI bleed, 81 mg aspirin with twice-daily administration of a PPI should be used[17].

Lipid-lowering therapy

No specific trials with lipid-lowering agents have been conducted in patients with CSA. Nevertheless, in the Scandinavian Simvastatin Survival Study (4S Study), many patients had CSA and experienced a reduction in angina as well as in major CAD events[17]. In addition, most of the major statin therapy randomized, controlled trials have demonstrated a decrease in revascularization requirements in patients on the active drug, clearly suggestive of a decrease in chest pain during the study. In the Medical Research Council/British Heart Foundation (MRC/BHF) Heart Protection Study of 20,536 patients >55 years old and with a history of known vascular disease including coronary disease, diabetes, or a major cardiovascular risk factor and a fasting total cholesterol level >135 mg/dl, fixed dose simvastatin (40 mg) resulted in a significant reduction in total mortality, vascular morbidity, and the need for revascularization procedures[18]. The benefits of simvastatin were seen across all subgroups, including both men and women, and in the elderly, and it was equally effective irrespective of baseline LDL levels, which in many patients were <100 mg/dl. Current guidelines recommend a target fasting LDL cholesterol level of <100 mg/dl in patients with CSA[11]. The most recent NCEP-ATP III directive suggests a target of <70 mg/dl for high-risk CAD patients[19].

In men with known CAD, and a HDL <40 mg/dl and LDL <130 mg/dl, treatment with gemfibrozil has been shown to reduce cardiovascular mortality and morbidity[20]. However, gemfibrozil should generally not be prescribed with a statin. Fenofibrate is the recommended fibrate for use with a statin. It should be noted that combination treatment with a statin and fibrates or nicotinic acid has not been adequately studied in patients with CSA and there are no outcome studies evaluating the beneficial effects of this combination therapy. Importantly, combination therapy should be used with caution because of a higher incidence of rhabdomyolysis.

Treatment of hypertension

Aggressive lowering of blood pressure, to a level of <135/85 mmHg in patients with hypertension and to <120/80 mmHg in those with diabetes mellitus, is the current recommendation. It has been shown that lowering blood pressure can reduce stroke rates by 40–52% and cardiovascular morbidity by 18–20%[21].

Angiotensin-converting enzyme inhibitors

Angiotensin-converting enzyme (ACE) inhibitors are recommended for use in all CSA patients who have suffered an MI. In addition, ACE inhibitors should be prescribed for patients with CSA who have diabetes mellitus, hypertension, proteinuria, chronic renal disease, or those with impaired LV

systolic function (LVEF <40%). In older patients, routine use of ACE inhibitors has been recommended based on the evidence provided by the positive results of the HOPE and EUROPA trials[22]. However, in patients with documented CAD and an LVEF >40%, ACE inhibitors have no proven benefit[23]. Therefore, there is room for disagreement regarding routine ACE inhibitor therapy in CSA patients who have not had an MI, are diabetic, have proteinuria or chronic renal disease, or have an LVEF <40%.

β-blockers

β-blockers improve survival and reduce the need for hospitalization in heart failure patients with an LVEF <40% and in survivors of acute MI. These drugs should thus be used as first-line therapy in patients with CSA who have reduced LV systolic function, provided that such patients are on background treatment with ACE inhibitors and are not in decompensated heart failure. Practice guidelines recommend that β-blockers are the first choice of therapy for uncomplicated CSA[2,11,13].

Exercise training

Patients with CSA should be encouraged to exercise 4–5 times per week to their anginal threshold. Exercise and other forms of lifestyle modification have become critical components of the overall wellbeing of patients with CSA.

Pharmacologic therapy

The primary consideration in the choice of pharmacologic agents for the treatment of angina should be to improve prognosis. Aspirin and lipid-lowering therapy have been shown to reduce the risk of death and nonfatal MI in both primary and secondary prevention trials. These data strongly suggest that cardiac events will also be reduced among patients with chronic stable angina.

The ACC/AHA guidelines suggest that aspirin (75–325 mg daily) should be routinely given to all patients without contraindications; clopidogrel can be used in those in whom aspirin is absolutely contraindicated[2].

Two landmark trials, the Cholesterol and Recurrent Events (CARE) Trial and Scandinavian Simvastatin Survival Study (4S) have established the benefit of aggressive lipid-lowering therapy for most patients with CAD, even when LDL levels are within the range considered acceptable for patients in a primary prevention setting[24,25]. In addition, the Medical Research Council/British Heart Foundation (MRC/BHF) Heart

Protection Study conducted in 20,536 high-risk adults with evidence of vascular disease or diabetes mellitus, showed that adding simvastatin 40 mg to existing therapies reduced the rates of MI, stroke, or revascularization by approximately 24%[26]. The benefit was seen regardless of age, gender, baseline lipid levels, or concomitant treatments for CAD. Importantly, this larger study refuted the CARE hypothesis that there was a threshold below which LDL lowering was ineffective. Based on these findings, it was estimated that simvastatin given for 5 years would protect 70–100 patients per 1,000 from experiencing a secondary event.

ACE inhibitors are recommended for all patients with CAD and for asymptomatic patients with CAD who also have diabetes or LV systolic dysfunction. The rationale for their use is based on the central role played by the renin–angiotensin system in maintaining endothelial integrity. The results of the Heart Outcomes Prevention Evaluation (HOPE) Trial showed that use of the tissue-specific ACE inhibitor, ramipril (10 mg/day), reduced the composite risk of cardiovascular death, MI, and stroke by approximately 25% in patients at high risk for, or with established, vascular disease in the absence of heart failure, regardless of age, gender, or coexisting disease[27]. A substudy of the HOPE trial also showed that ACE inhibitors prevent overt nephropathy and other microvascular outcomes in patients with type 1 or type 2 diabetes[28].

On the basis of their potentially beneficial effects on morbidity and mortality, β-blockers should be strongly considered as initial therapy for CSA, as secondary prevention in post-MI patients, and as a means of reducing morbidity and mortality among patients with hypertension, provided that there is no major contraindication including a risk of asthma/bronchospasm. Diabetes mellitus is not a contraindication to their use[2].

Long-acting or slow-release CCBs are indicated to relieve symptoms in patients with CSA, and they do so without enhancing the risk of adverse cardiac events. They are often preferable to long-acting nitrates for maintenance therapy because of their sustained effects[2]. Short-acting nitrates do not lose their effect on symptom relief, but long-acting nitrates may produce tolerance.

Revascularization

Revascularization is indicated for patients with: (1) CSA and 3-vessel disease, (2) 2-vessel disease with proximal left anterior descending artery involvement, (3) 1- or 2-vessel disease with a large area of viable myocardium and high-risk criteria on noninvasive testing, (4) significant (>50%) left main stem stenosis, (5) and with refractory symptoms, and (6) for improving quality of life[2]. In asymptomatic patients, the same recommendations apply, although the aim is to improve prognosis[2].

Surgical procedures, which are invasive and costly and carry with them a significant degree of morbidity and mortality, are nevertheless a very effective mechanical means

---

Table 6.18 Candidates for PCI

Indications for coronary angioplasty (class 1)
Clinical
- Myocardial ischemia during laboratory testing (must be severe if symptoms are absent)
- Resuscitation from cardiac arrest or from sustained ventricular tachycardia in the absence of acute MI
- Undergoing high-risk noncardiac surgery
- Angina pectoris inadequately responsive to medical therapy
- Within 6 hours (or 12 hours if symptoms persist) of acute MI
- Unstable or post-MI angina
- Cardiogenic shock within 12 hours of symptoms

Angiographic
- Lesion(s) believed to be amenable to angioplasty and of low risk for morbidity or mortality; if very symptomatic, a moderate likelihood of success is acceptable
- In cases of multi-vessel disease, nearly complete or complete revascularization is possible

of restoring adequate myocardial perfusion (*Table 6.17*). Coronary angioplasty with stenting also offers an effective mechanical therapeutic modality, although repeat procedures are required because of restenosis (*Tables 6.18–6.20*). *Table 6.20* summarizes results from the two pivotal randomized trials of stenting versus balloon

angioplasty. Although the patient subsets and enrolling countries were different, the results were concordant. The goal of the US initiated STRESS trial was to compare the effects of stent placement and standard balloon angioplasty on angiographically detected restenosis and clinical outcomes. Palmaz-Schatz stents were used. Patients who underwent stenting had a higher rate of procedural success than those who underwent standard balloon angioplasty (96.1% *vs.* 89.6%, $p = 0.011$), a larger immediate increase in the diameter of the lumen (1.72 +/- 0.46 mm *vs.* 1.23 +/- 0.48 mm, $p<0.001$), and a larger luminal diameter immediately after the procedure (2.49 +/- 0.43 mm *vs.* 1.99 +/- 0.47 mm, $p<0.001$). At 6 months, the patients with stented lesions continued to have a larger luminal diameter (1.74 +/- 0.60 mm *vs.* 1.56 +/- 0.65 mm, $p = 0.007$) and a lower rate of restenosis (31.6% *vs.* 42.1%, $p = 0.046$) than those treated with balloon angioplasty. There were no coronary events (death; MI; coronary-artery bypass surgery; vessel closure, including stent thrombosis; or repeated angioplasty) in 80.5% of the patients in the stent group and 76.2% of those in the angioplasty group ($p = 0.16$). Revascularization of the original target lesion because of recurrent myocardial ischemia was performed less frequently in the stent group than in the angioplasty group (10.2% *vs.* 15.4%, $p = 0.06$). The investigators concluded that in selected patients, placement of an intracoronary stent, as compared with balloon angioplasty, results in an improved rate of procedural success, a lower rate of angiographically detected restenosis, a similar rate of clinical events after 6 months, and a less frequent need for revascularization of the original coronary lesion.

Table 6.19 Contraindications to PCI

Absolute
- No significant lesion (<50%)
- Unprotected significant stenosis of the left main coronary artery (>50%)
- No surgical program within the institution

Relative
- Significant coagulopathy
- Diffusely diseased saphenous vein grafts without focal lesion
- Diffusely diseased native vessels (suitable for bypass)
- Only remaining artery to the myocardium
- Chronic total occlusion
- Borderline significant stenosis (usually ≥50%)
- Stenosis of a noninfarct-related artery during acute myocardial infarction

Table 6.20 Randomized trials of PTCA *vs.* stent replacement (in-hospital outcome)

Event	Stress trial (n = 410)			Benestent trial (n = 520)		
	Stent (%)	PTCA (%)	P value	Stent (%)	PTCA (%)	P value
Clinical success	96.1	89.6	<0.01	92.7	91.1	-
Death	1.5	0	-	0	0	-
Q-wave MI	3.0	2.9	-	1.9	0.8	-
Abrupt closure	3.4	1.5	-	2.7	3.5	-
Emergency CABG	2.4	4.0	-	9	1.6	-
Major bleed/vascular complication	7.3	4.0	-	13	3.1	<0.001
Any event	5.9	7.9	-	6.9	6.2	-

In the European-initiated BENESTENT trial, the primary clinical endpoints were death, the occurrence of a cerebrovascular accident, MI, the need for coronary artery bypass surgery, or a second percutaneous intervention involving the previously treated lesion, either at the time of the initial procedure or during the subsequent 7 months. The primary angiographic endpoint was the minimal luminal diameter at follow-up, as determined by quantitative coronary angiography. After exclusions, 52 patients in the stent group (20%) and 76 patients in the angioplasty group (30%) reached a primary clinical endpoint (RR 0.68; 95% CI 0.50–0.92; $p = 0.02$). The difference in clinical event rates was explained mainly by a reduced need for a second coronary angioplasty in the stent group (RR 0.58; 95% CI 0.40–0.85; $p = 0.005$). The mean (+/- SD) minimal luminal diameters immediately after the procedure were 2.48 +/- 0.39 mm in the stent group and 2.05 +/- 0.33 mm in the angioplasty group; at follow-up, the diameters were 1.82 +/- 0.64 mm in the stent group and 1.73 +/- 0.55 mm in the angioplasty group ($p = 0.09$), which correspond to rates of restenosis (diameter of stenosis, ≥50%) of 22% and 32%, respectively ($p = 0.02$). Peripheral vascular complications necessitating surgery, blood transfusion, or both were more frequent after stenting than after balloon angioplasty (13.5% *vs.* 3.1%, $p<0.001$). The mean hospital stay was significantly longer in the stent group than in the angioplasty group (8.5 *vs.* 3.1 days, $p<0.001$).

Thus, the clinical and angiographic outcomes were better in patients who received a stent than in those who received standard coronary angioplasty. However, this benefit was achieved at the cost of a significantly higher risk of vascular complications at the access site and a longer hospital stay.

Drug-eluting stents (DESs), which are coated with slow-release anti-proliferative and immunosuppressant drugs, have been dramatically effective in reducing the incidence of restenosis. Clinical studies with a sirolimus-coated stent have shown a reduction in restenosis of 91% compared with a bare metal stent (3.2% *vs.* 35.4%, respectively)[29]. Other studies evaluating stents coated with paclitaxel, actinomycin, and tacrolimus have reported varying degrees of success[30]. However, the troubling, albeit uncommon phenomenon of late stent thrombosis seen with DESs makes long-term combination anti-platelet therapy and close follow-up imperative.

These factors and challenges highlight the need for developing strategies and interventions that can induce plaque regression and/or stabilization, thereby reversing the disease process itself. The fact that asymptomatic patients comprise a target population for this type of approach highlights the need for cost-effective methods for screening the general population for 'silent' risk factors that predispose to atherosclerotic disease in later life.

Patients who have refractory angina despite optimal medical therapy (*Tables 6.21, 6.22*) and are not candidates

---

Table 6.21 Definition of refractory angina pectoris

- Persistence of severe anginal symptoms (class III + IV) despite maximally tolerated conventional anti-anginal combination therapy
- Not suitable for percutaneous or surgical revascularization

(Adapted from Frazier OH, *et al.* Myocardial revascularization with laser. Preliminary findings. *Circulation* 1995;**92**:1158–1165; Leschke M, *et al. J Am Coll Cardiol* 1996;**27**:575–584; Jessurun GA, *et al. Cort Art Dis* 1997;**8**:33–38.)

Table 6.22 Clinical characteristics of refractory angina pectoris

- Severe coronary insufficiency but only moderately impaired LV function
- 3-vessel coronary artery disease with diffuse atherosclerosis
- Have had >1 MI
- 70% have undergone previous CABG

(Adapted from Frazier OH, *et al.* Myocardial revascularization with laser. Preliminary findings. *Circulation* 1995;**92**:1158–1165; Leschke M, *et al. J Am Coll Cardiol* 1996;**27**:575–584; Jessurun GA, *et al. Cort Art Dis* 1997;**8**:33–38.)

Table 6.23 Management of nonrevascularizable chest pain

- Long-term intermittent urokinase therapy
- Neurostimulation
- TENS
- SCS
- Sequential external counterpulsation (SECP)
- Chelation therapy
- Therapeutic angiogenesis
- Transmyocardial laser revascularization

Table 6.24 Protocol for enhanced external counterpulsation for angina

- Timed, sequential pneumatic inflation of lower extremity cuffs during diastole
- Augments diastolic pressure (increased coronary perfusion)
- ?Facilitated collateral development and enhanced collateral perfusion
- Increased venous return
- Decreased ventricular afterload 1 hour per day, 5x/week for 7 weeks (35 treatments)

(From Lawson WE, Hui JC, Soroff JS, *et al*. Efficacy of enhanced external counterpulsation in the treatment of angina pectoris. *Am J Cardiol* 1992;**70**:859–862; Lawson WE, Hui JC, Zheng ZS, *et al*. Three-year sustained benefit from enhanced external counterpulsation in chronic angina pectoris. *Am J Cardiol* 1995;**75**:840–841; Lawson WE, Hui JC, Zheng ZS, *et al*. Can angiographic findings predict which coronary patients will benefit from enhanced external counterpulsation? *Am J Cardiol* 1996;**77**:1107–1109.)

for revascularization procedures, may be candidates for some new techniques (*Table 6.23*)[31]. Such a technique is enhanced external counterpulsation (EECP) (*Table 6.24, 6.6*). In a number of small nonrandomized clinical studies there has been significant symptomatic improvement, improvement in exercise capacity, and improvement in perfusion defects (80%). Rather surprisingly, the beneficial effect is durable for up to 3 years. The benefit appears to be inversely related to the extent of CAD. In assessing the suitability of patients for this form of therapy, transmission

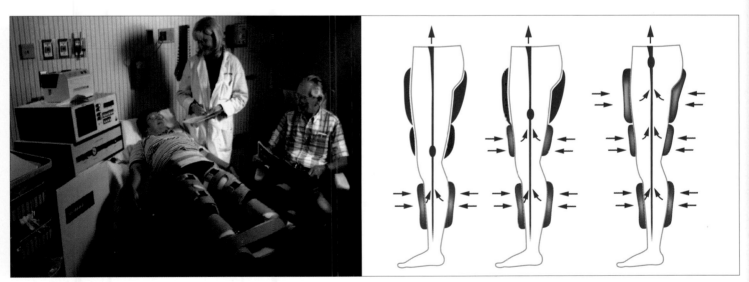

6.6 The EECP procedure. A series of three cuffs are wrapped around the calves, lower thighs, and upper thighs and buttocks: there is sequential distal to proximal compression upon diastole, simultaneous release of pressure at end-diastole, and increased diastolic pressure and retrograde aortic flow. This produces increased venous return and systolic unloading, resulting in increased cardiac output.

Table 6.25 Summary of MUST-EECP results

Compared to sham, EECP
- Increased time to exercise-induced ST segment depression ($p = 0.01$)
- Decreased the frequency of angina episodes ($p<0.04$)

Compared to baseline
- Exercise duration increased significantly in both groups (sham $p<0.03$, active $p<0.001$)
- Time to ST segment depression increased significantly in active group only ($p<0.002$)

EECP was generally well tolerated but with significantly fewer adverse experiences reported in the sham group

Table 6.26 Protocol for TENS treatment of angina

- Two cutaneous electrodes, one in the dermatome with the highest intensity of projected pain and the other in the contralateral dermatome
- Intensity of stimulation adjusted below the individual pain threshold
- Stimulation given for 1 hour at least 3x/day and for duration of angina plus 10 minutes

(Adapted from Mannheimer C, *et al*. Influence of naloxone on the effects of high frequency transcutaneous electrical nerve stimulation in angina pectoris induced by atrial pacing. *Br Heart J* 1989;**62**:36–42; De Jongste MJ, *et al*. Stimulation characteristics, complications and efficacy of spinal cord stimulation systems in patients with refractory angina: a prospective feasibility study. *PACE* 1994;**17**:1751–1760.)

Table 6.27 Protocol for SCS treatment of angina

- Implantation of uni/bipolar electrode at T1 or T2 level and stimulator in a subcutaneous pocket in upper abdomen with telemetric manipulation (re-op necessary after approximately 4 years)
- Results in reduction in ischemic burden, episodes of ischemia and quality of life (QOL)
- Improved exercise duration, time to angina, ST depression and improved perfusion

(Adapted from Romano M, *et al*. Technical and clinical problems in patients with simultaneous implantation of a cardiac pacemaker and spinal cord stimulator. *PACE* 1993;**16**:1639–1644; De Jongste MJ, *et al*. Efficacy of spinal cord stimulation as adjuvant therapy for intractable angina pectoris; a prospective randomized clinical study. *J Am Coll Cardiol* 1994;**23**:1592–1597.)

of diastolic pressure and volume to the distal vessel appears to require a patent proximal conduit[32–34]. The exact mechanism of benefit of EECP remains unclear. In patients showing some but not full improvement after 35 treatments, a further 10 treatments have been shown to provide additional benefit. *Table 6.25* summarizes the Multicenter Study of (MUST) -EECP clinical results. In most patients, EECP reduces anginal pain, increases functional ability, and improves quality of life, both short- and long-term.

Transcutaneous electrical nerve stimulation (TENS) and spinal cord stimulation (SCS) reduce the adrenergic state by stimulating at high frequency large myelinated type A fibers which inhibit impulse transmission through smaller type C fibers and reduce activation of central pain receptors. There is also a direct sympatholytic effect, with stimulation of dorsal roots leading to segmental reflexes that induce inhibition of tonic sympathetic activity (*Tables 6.26, 6.27*)[35,36]. Neurostimulation delays rather than abolishes the occurrence of angina as a warning signal for ischemia, thus does not conceal the pain of ACS[37,38].

The feasibility of carbon dioxide (CO_2) laser radiation to create transmyocardial revascularization (TMR) in dogs was first reported by Mirhoseini and Cayton[40]. Subsequent experimental studies showed patent channels at 1 month and 12 months with endothelialization and no scar tissue. In addition, other studies showed no effect on collateral myocardial blood flow or infarct size after coronary occlusion. In humans, immediate relief of angina after TMR was observed in early trials, with success rates reported as high as 80%. The proposed mechanism of benefit of TMR includes: (1) creation of channels with improved perfusion, (2) cardiomyocyte denervation, (3) angiogenesis, and (4) placebo effect. It was expected that the benefit would dissipate after 6 months but 50% of patients benefit up to 3 years. The most likely mechanism appears to be cardiomyocyte denervation, but the exact mechanism remains unclear. However, no beneficial effects were reported in randomized controlled trials and this therapy has fallen out of favor.

References

1 Murray CJ, Lopez AD. Alternative projections of mortality and disability by cause 1990–2020: Global Burden of Disease Study. *Lancet* 1997;**349**:1498–1504.

2 American College of Cardiology/American Heart Association Task Force on Practice Guidelines (Committee on the Management of Patients with Chronic Stable Angina). ACC/AHA 2002 guideline update for the management of patients with chronic stable angina – summary article. *J Am Coll Cardiol* 2003;**41**:159–168.

3 Sackett DL, Haynes RB, Guyatt GH, Tugwell P. *Clinical Epidemiology: A Basic Science for Clinical Medicine*. Little, Brown and Company, Boston, 1991, p. 20.

4 Pryor DB, Shaw L, McCants CB, *et al.* Value of the history and physical in identifying patients at increased risk for coronary artery disease. *Ann Intern Med* 1993;**118**:81–90.

5 Lewington S, Clarke R, Qizilbash N, Peto R, Collins R. Age-specific relevance of usual blood pressure to vascular mortality: a meta-analysis of individual data for one million adults in 61 prospective studies. *Lancet* 2002;**360**:1903–1913.

6 Diamond GA, Forrester JS. Analysis of probability as an aid in the clinical diagnosis of coronary artery disease. *N Engl J Med* 1979;**300**:81–90, 1350–1358.

7 Stuart RJ, Ellestad MH. National survey of exercise stress testing facilities. *Chest* 1980;**77**:94–97.

8 Gibbons RJ, Balady GJ, Bricker JT, *et al.* ACC/AHA 2002 guideline update for exercise testing: a report of the American College of Cardiology/American Heart Association Task Force on Practice Guidelines (Committee on Exercise Testing). *Circulation* 2002;**106**:1883–1892.

9 Daly C, Clemens F, Lopez-Sendon JL, *et al.* on behalf of the Euro Heart Survey Investigators. The impact of guideline compliant medical therapy on clinical outcome in patients with stable angina: findings from the Euro Heart Survey of stable angina. *Europ Heart J* 2006;**27**:1298–1304.

10 Ezzati M, Lopez AD, Rodgers A, Vander Hoorn S, Murray CJ. Selected major risk factors and global and regional burden of disease. *Lancet* 2002;**360**:1347–1360.

11 Thadani U. Current medical management of chronic stable angina. *J Cardiovasc Pharmacol Ther* 2004;**9**(suppl 1):S11–S29.

12 Task Force of the European Society of Cardiology. Management of stable angina pectoris: recommendations of the Task Force of the European Society of Cardiology. *Eur Heart J* 1997;**18**:394–413.

13 Abrams J. Chronic stable angina. *N Engl J Med* 2005;**352**:2524–2533.

14 Davies MJ, Thomas AC. Plaque fissuring: the cause of acute myocardial infarction, sudden ischemic death, and crescendo angina. *Br Heart J* 1985;**53**:363–368.

15 Doll R, Peto R. Mortality in relation to smoking: 20-years' observations on male British doctors. *BMJ* 1976;**2**:1526–1536.

16 Juul-Moller S, Edvardson N, Jahnmatz B, Rosen A, Sorensen S, Omblus R, for SAPAT (Swedish Angina Pectoris Aspirin Trial) Group. Double blind trial of aspirin in primary prevention of myocardial infarction in patients with stable chronic angina pectoris. *Lancet* 1992;**340**:1421–1425.

17 Chan FKL, Ching JYL, Hung LCT, *et al.* Clopidogrel versus aspirin and esomeprazole to prevent recurrent ulcer bleeding. *N Engl J Med* 2005;**352**:238–244.

18 MRC/BHF Heart Protection Study of cholesterol lowering with simvastatin in high risk individuals: a randomized placebo controlled trial. *Lancet* 2003;**36**:7–22.

19 Grundy SM, Cleeman JI, Merz CN, *et al.*, for the Coordinating Committee of the National Cholesterol Education Program. Implications of recent clinical trials for the National Cholesterol Education Program: Adult Treatment Panel guidelines. *Circulation* 2004;**110**:227–239.

20 Rubins HB, Robins S, Collins D, *et al.* Gemfibrozil for the secondary prevention of coronary heart disease in men with low levels of high-density lipoprotein cholesterol. *N Engl J Med* 1999;**341**:410–418.

21 Chobanian AV, Bakris GL, Black HR, *et al.*, and the National High Blood Pressure Education Program Coordinating Committee. The seventh report of the Joint National Committee on Prevention, Detection, Evaluation and Treatment of High Blood Pressure: the JNC 7 Report. *JAMA* 2003;**289**:2560–2571.

22 European Trial on reduction of cardiac events with perindopril in stable artery disease investigation. Efficacy of perindopril reduction of cardiovascular events among patients with stable coronary artery disease: randomized, double-blind, placebo-controlled, multicenter trial (the EUROPA Study). *Lancet* 2003;**362**:782–789.

23 The PEACE Trial Investigators. Angiotensin-converting-enzyme inhibition in stable coronary artery disease. *N Engl J Med* 2004;**351**:2058–2068.

24 Randomized trial of cholesterol lowering in 4444 patients with coronary heart disease, the Scandinavian Simvastatin Survival Study (4S). *Lancet* 1994;**344**:1383–1389.

25 Sacks FM, Pfeffer MA, Moye LA, *et al.* The effect of pravastatin on coronary events after myocardial infarction in patients with average cholesterol levels: Cholesterol and Recurrent Events trial investigators. *N Engl J Med* 1996;**335**:1001–1009.

26 Heart Protection Study Collaborative Group, MRC/BHF Heart Protection Study of cholesterol lowering with simvastatin in 20,536 high-risk patients: a randomised placebo-controlled trial. *Lancet* 2002;**360**:7–22.

27 The Heart Outcomes Prevention Evaluation Study Investigators. Effects of an angiotensin-converting-enzyme inhibitor, ramipril, on cardiovascular events in high-risk patients. *N Engl J Med* 2000;**342**:145–153.

28 Heart Outcomes Prevention Evaluation (HOPE) Study Investigators. Effects of ramipril on cardiovascular and microvascular outcomes in people with diabetes mellitus: results of the HOPE study and MICRO-HOPE substudy. *Lancet* 2000;**355**:253–259.

29 Moses JW, Leon MB, Popma JJ, *et al.* A multicenter randomized clinical study of the Sirolimus-eluting stent in native coronary lesions: clinical outcomes. *Circulation* 2002;**106**:II-392.

30 Grube E, Gerckens U, Muller R, Bullesfield L. Drug eluting stents: initial experiences. *Z Kardiol* 2002;**91**(suppl 3):44–48.

31 Kleiman NS, Patel NC, Allen KB, *et al.* Evolving revascularization approaches for myocardial ischemia. *Am J Cardiol* 2003;**92**(suppl):9N–17N.

32 Lawson WE, Hui JC, Soroff JS, *et al.* Efficacy of enhanced external counterpulsation in the treatment of angina pectoris. *Am J Cardiol* 1992;**70**:859–862.

33 Lawson WE, Hui JC, Zheng ZS, *et al.* Three-year sustained benefit from enhanced external counterpulsation in chronic angina pectoris. *Am J Cardiol* 1995;**75**:840–841.

34 Lawson WE, Hui JC, Zheng ZS, *et al.* Can angiographic findings predict which coronary patients will benefit from enhanced external counterpulsation? *Am J Cardiol* 1996;**77**:1107–1109.

35 Mannheimer C, Emanuelsson H, Waagstein F, Wilhelmsson C. Influence of naloxone on the effects of high frequency transcutaneous electrical nerve stimulation in angina pectoris induced by atrial pacing. *Br Heart J* 1989;**62**:36–42.

36 De Jongste MJ, Nagelkerke D, Hoovschuur CM, *et al.* Stimulation characteristics, complications and efficacy of spinal cord stimulation systems in patients with refractory angina: a prospective feasibility study. *PACE* 1994;**17**:1751–1760.

37 Romano M, Zucco F, Baldini MR, Allaria B. Technical and clinical problems in patients with simultaneous implantation of a cardiac pacemaker and spinal cord stimulator. *PACE* 1993;**16**:1639–1644.

38 De Jongste MJ, Hautvast RW, Hillege HL, Lie KI. Efficacy of spinal cord stimulation as adjuvant therapy for intractable angina pectoris; a prospective randomized clinical study. *J Am Coll Cardiol* 1994;**23**:1592–1597.

39 Mirhoseini M, Shelgikars S, Cayton M. Transmyocardial laser revascularization: a review. *J Clin Laser Med Surg* 1993;**11**:15–19.

Index

nociceptors 10
noncardiac disease *9*
noninvasive evaluation 29–30, 77–8
  patient and test selection 30
  special populations 47
  strategy 46
noninvasive testing, *see also individual
  evaluation methods*
nuclear imaging 30, 34–6

obesity 59, 62
Olmsted County study 2
outcomes of CAD 2, *2*

paclitaxel 94
pain, *see* chest pain
Palmaz-Schatz stents 93
pathophysiology 3–10
percutaneous transluminal coronary
  angioplasty (PTCA) 87–9, *88, 89*
  comparison with medical therapy
    87–9, *88*
  contraindications 93
  recurrence of angina 89
  restenosis after 93–4, *93*
pericarditis 16
peripheral pulses 20
physical examination 19–20, *19*
plaque, atherosclerotic, *see* atheroma
polypharmacy 79
positron emission tomography (PET)
  37
pre-excitation syndrome 34
pre-test probability 13, 20, *22–3*
precipitating factors 14
precordial palpation *19*, 20
Prinzmetal's angina 68
Prospective Studies Collaboration 80
proton pump inhibitors (PPIs) 90
psychiatric conditions 17, *17*
pulmonary conditions, causing chest
  pain 16, *16*

radiation exposure, CT imaging 44, 47
radionuclide perfusion testing 34–6, 37
ramipril 92
Raynaud's phenomenon *68*

recurrence of angina
  after revascularization 89, *89*
  see also refractory angina
refractory angina *79*, 94–5
  characteristics *94*
  definition *94*
relieving factors 14
renal failure *57*, 58
renal toxicity, contrast agents 58
restenosis 93–4, *93, 94*
revascularization, *see* coronary artery
  revascularization
right coronary artery (RCA)
  aneurysm 72, 73
  angiography 51, 52, *53*, 65, 66
  complete occlusion 26
  MSCT angiography 45
risk factors 18, *19*
  modification 79–80
  vascular 77
risk stratification 77–8

Scandinavian Simvastatin Survival
  Study (4S Study) 90–1, *91–2*
serum markers 27–9, 75, 78
simvastatin 90–1
single photon emission computed
  tomography (SPECT) 30, 34, 35, 37
smoking 68, *68*
  cessation 90
  coronary vasospasm 68–9
sodium bicarbonate 58
spinal cord stimulation (SCS) *96*, 97
statin therapy 90–1
stent placement 89, 93, *93*
stents, drug-eluting (DESs) 89, 94
stress testing
  echocardiography 38–9
  exercise EKG 30–4, 47
  magnetic resonance imaging 42, 43
  pharmacological 34–6
STRESS trial 93
sudden cardiac death 6, 70, 77
surgery
  noncardiac 47
  see also coronary artery bypass
    grafting (CABG)

survival rates 2
symptoms
  correlation with atherosclerosis 55,
    55
  other than chest pain (angina-
    equivalents) 14
  see also chest pain
syndrome X, cardiac 69

tachycardia 19, 75
tachypnea 19
tacrolimus 94
three vessel coronary disease 35, 43, 55
thromboembolism, coronary 71–2
Thrombosis in Myocardial Infarction
  (TIMI) score 30, 64, *65*, 66
tobacco use, *see* smoking
transcutaneous electrical nerve
  stimulation (TENS) *96*, 97
transmyocardial revascularization
  (TMR) 97
triglycerides, total serum 80
troponins, *see* cardiac troponins

ultrasound, intravascular 58, 59, 62, *63*

variant (Prinzmetal's) angina 68–9
vascular bruits 20
vasoconstriction 8
vasodilating agents 36, 60
ventricular ectopy 32, 33
ventricular fibrillation 6
verapamil 87
vital signs 19, *19*

wall motion
  abnormalities 38, 42
  assessment 42
women 2, 47
World Health Organization (WHO) 77

xanthelasma 20
xanthomas 20